AF879881

It's easy to get lost in the cancer world

Let NCCN Guidelines for Patients® be your guide

- ✓ Step-by-step guides to the cancer care options likely to have the best results
- ✓ Based on treatment guidelines used by health care providers worldwide
- ✓ Designed to help you discuss cancer treatment with your doctors

National Comprehensive Cancer Network®

NCCN Guidelines for Patients® are developed by the National Comprehensive Cancer Network® (NCCN®)

NCCN

- An alliance of leading cancer centers across the United States devoted to patient care, research, and education

Cancer centers that are part of NCCN: NCCN.org/cancercenters

NCCN Clinical Practice Guidelines in Oncology (NCCN Guidelines®)

- Developed by doctors from NCCN cancer centers using the latest research and years of experience
- For providers of cancer care all over the world
- Expert recommendations for cancer screening, diagnosis, and treatment

Free online at NCCN.org/guidelines

NCCN Guidelines for Patients

- Present information from the NCCN Guidelines in an easy-to-learn format
- For people with cancer and those who support them
- Explain the cancer care options likely to have the best results

Free online at NCCN.org/patientguidelines

NATIONAL COMPREHENSIVE CANCER NETWORK FOUNDATION
Guiding Treatment. Changing Lives.

and supported by funding from NCCN Foundation®

These NCCN Guidelines for Patients are based on the NCCN Guidelines® for Pancreatic Cancer, Version 2.2021 – February 25, 2021.

NCCN Foundation seeks to support the millions of patients and their families affected by a cancer diagnosis by funding and distributing NCCN Guidelines for Patients. NCCN Foundation is also committed to advancing cancer treatment by funding the nation's promising doctors at the center of innovation in cancer research. For more details and the full library of patient and caregiver resources, visit NCCN.org/patients.

National Comprehensive Cancer Network (NCCN) / NCCN Foundation
3025 Chemical Road, Suite 100
Plymouth Meeting, PA 19462
215.690.0300

Supporters

Endorsed by

Hirshberg Foundation for Pancreatic Cancer Research

The Hirshberg Foundation for Pancreatic Cancer Research is focused on finding a cure for pancreatic cancer, and empowering the patients and families whose lives are touched by this disease. Founded in 1997, the foundation funds groundbreaking scientific research, provides patient education and support, and sustains hope that this cancer will be eradicated once and for all. pancreatic.org

Let's Win! Pancreatic Cancer

The NCCN Guidelines for Patients are the gold standard for pancreatic cancer treatment information. The guidelines provide comprehensive explanations of the disease, stages, and treatments options in language patients can understand. Let's Win! Pancreatic Cancer has included a link to the NCCN Pancreatic Cancer Patient Guidelines since our launch. letswinpc.org

Lustgarten Foundation

As the world's largest private funder of pancreatic cancer research, we are honored to endorse the NCCN Guidelines for Patients®: Pancreatic Cancer. Receiving a pancreatic cancer diagnosis is both overwhelming and life-altering for patients and their loved ones, and having the most up-to-date, comprehensive information contained in these guidelines is crucial for navigating through this disease. These NCCN Patient Guidelines are a valuable resource for helping everyone impacted by pancreatic cancer to better understand the disease, evaluate treatment options, and make informed decisions. lustgarten.org

Pancreatic Cancer Action Network (PanCAN)

As the organization taking bold action to improve the lives of everyone impacted by pancreatic cancer by advancing scientific research, building community, sharing knowledge, and advocating for patients, the Pancreatic Cancer Action Network (PanCAN) supports the NCCN Guidelines for Patients on pancreatic cancer. This evidence-based resource is a valuable tool to help patients talk to their healthcare team about the best options for treating and managing their disease. pancan.org

The National Pancreas Foundation

The National Pancreas Foundation provides hope for those suffering from pancreatitis and pancreatic cancer through funding cutting edge research, advocating for new and better therapies, and providing support and education for patients, caregivers, and health care professionals. pancreasfoundation.org

With generous support from

Ken & Lisa Ganiszewski

To make a gift or learn more, please visit NCCNFoundation.org/donate or e-mail PatientGuidelines@nccn.org.

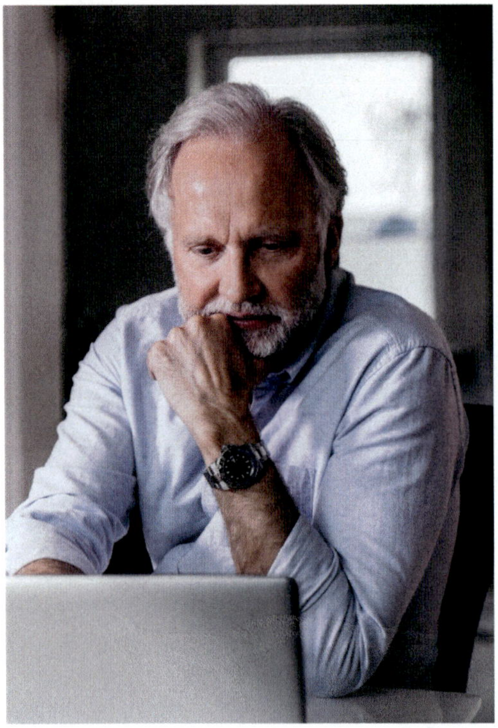
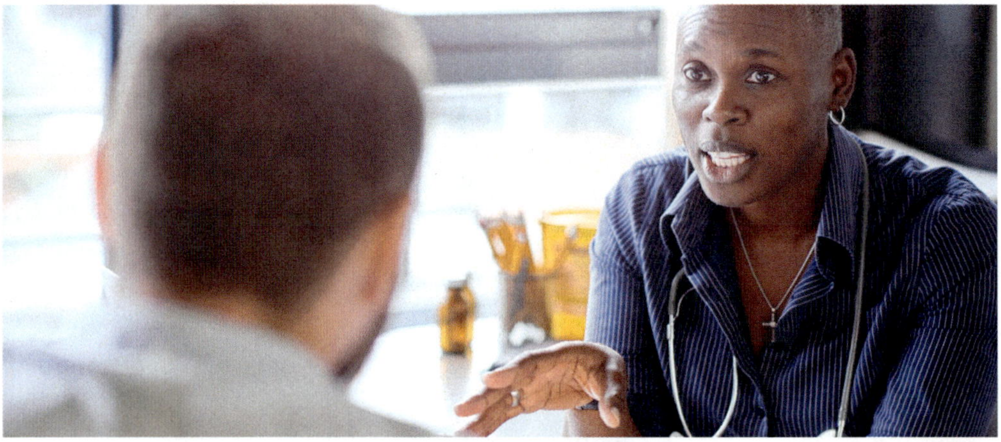
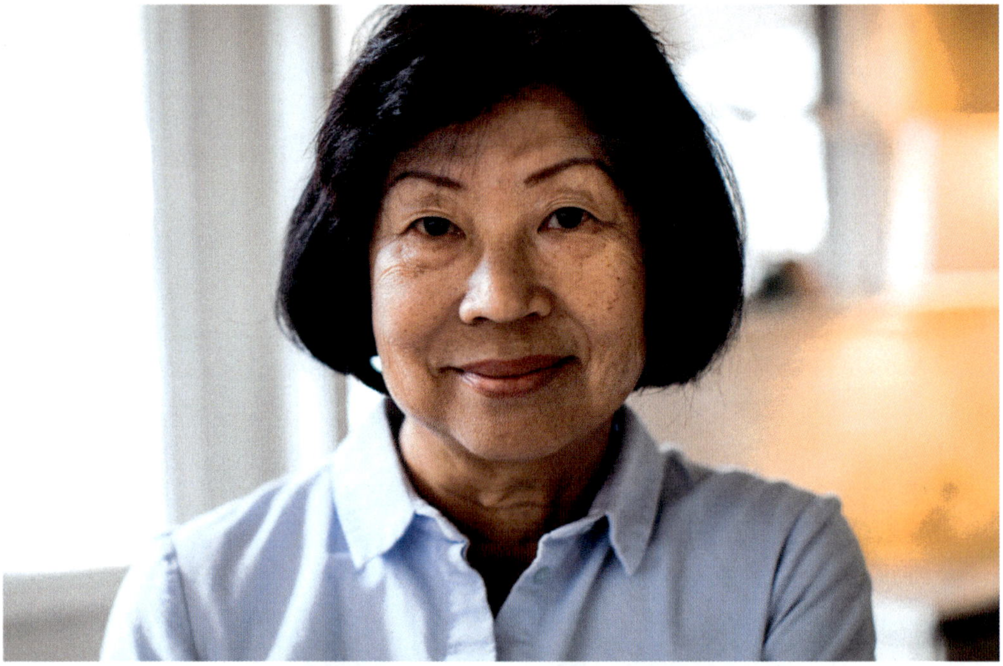
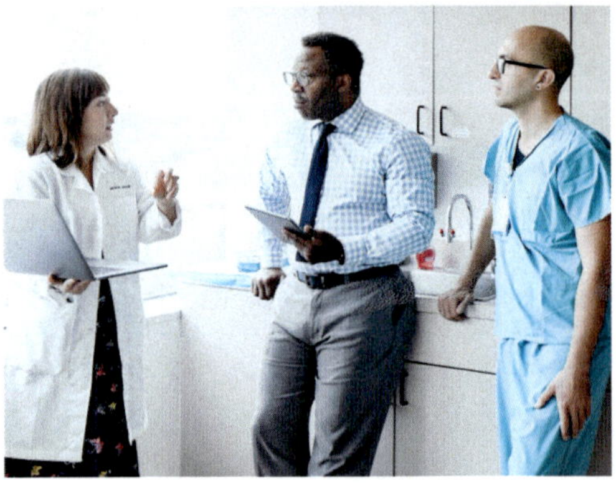
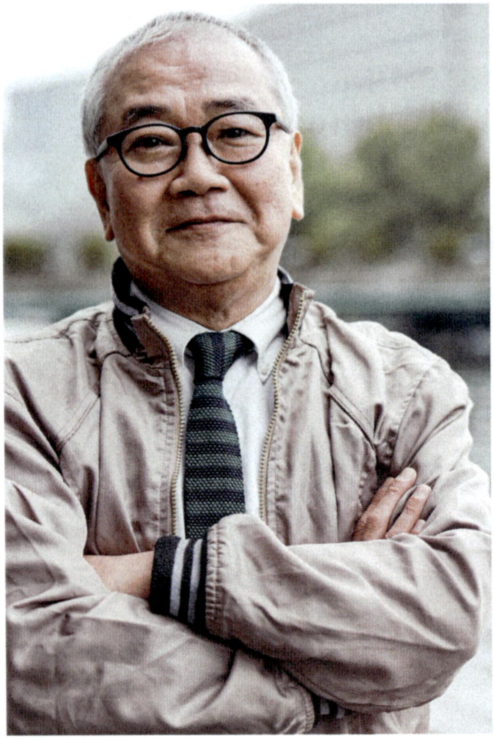
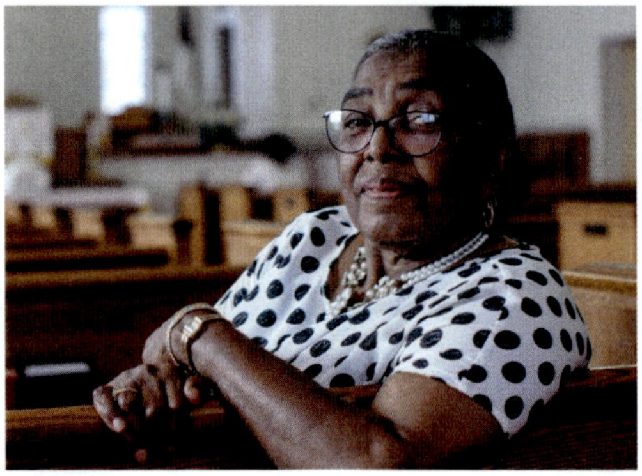
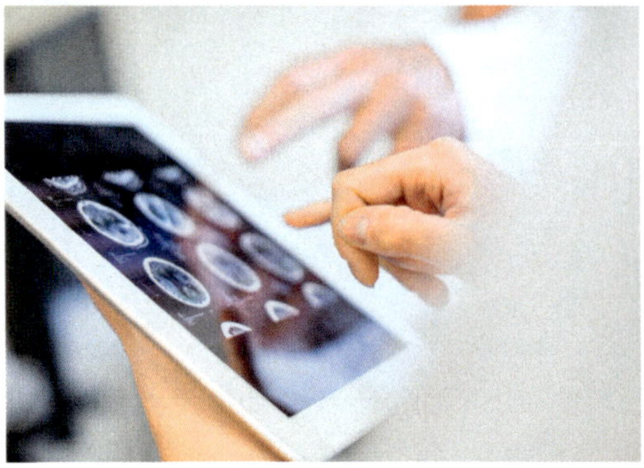
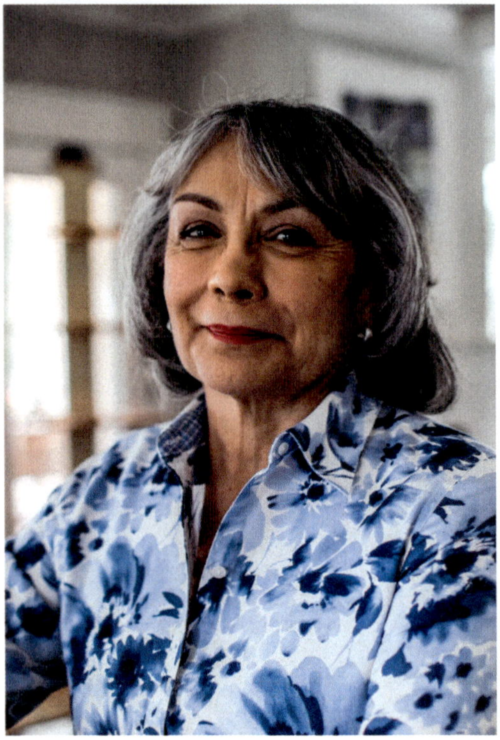

Contents

1 Pancreatic cancer basics

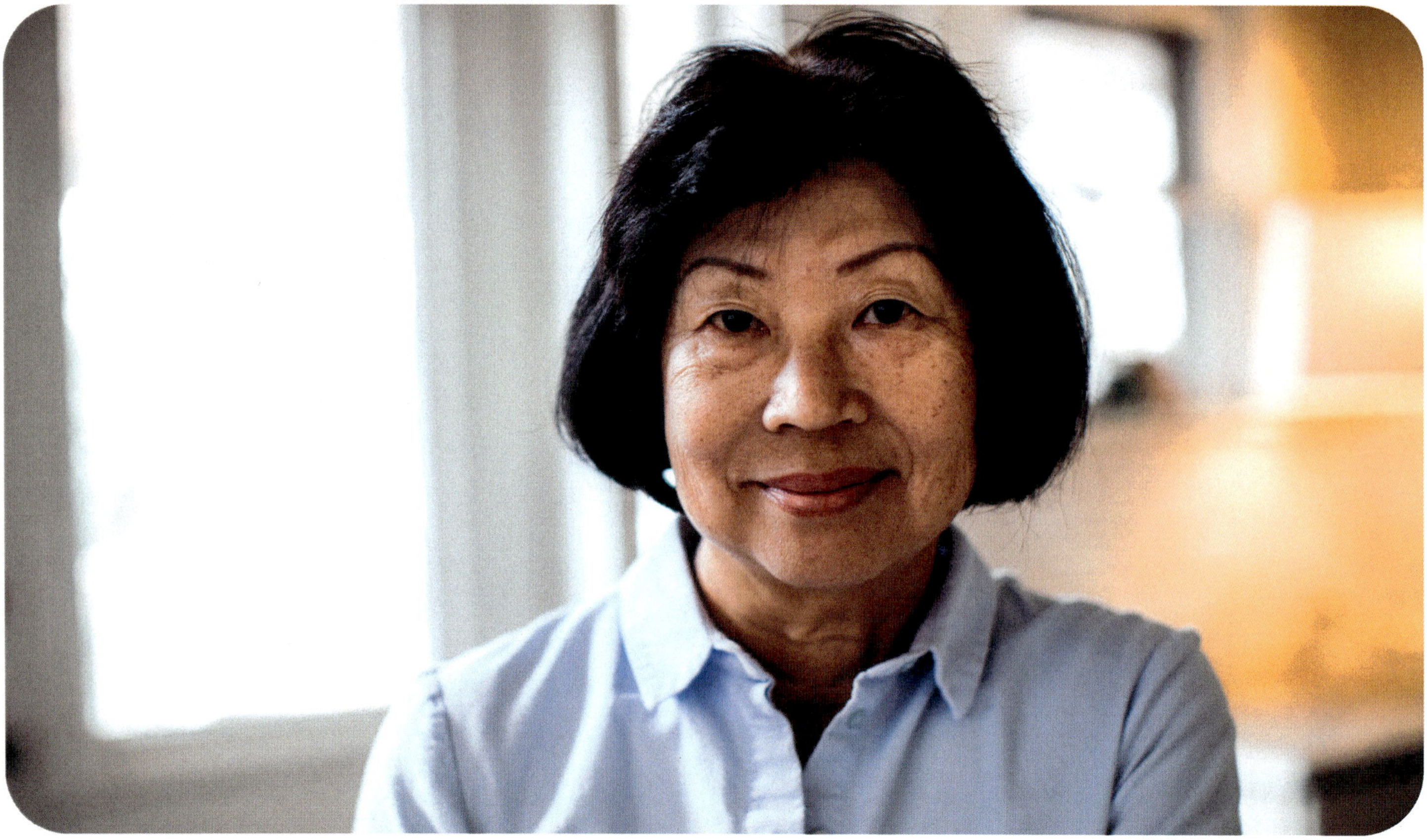

The pancreas is a large gland found in the abdomen behind the stomach. It helps digest food and control blood sugar. This chapter will discuss the pancreas and provide an overview of pancreatic cancer.

The pancreas

The pancreas is a large gland found in your abdomen. A gland is an organ that makes fluids or chemicals the body needs. The pancreas is about 6 inches long.

The pancreas lies behind the stomach and across the spine. The liver is located close to the pancreas, above the gallbladder. The small intestine is wrapped along the wide end of the pancreas. The spleen is found at the tail end of the pancreas.

The liver removes waste from blood and makes bile. Bile is a fluid that helps to digest food. The gallbladder stores bile from the liver. The common bile duct carries bile from the liver into the main pancreatic duct. From the main pancreatic duct, bile and enzymes empty into the duodenum. The duodenum is the first part of the small intestine, which absorbs nutrients from food you eat. The jejunum is the middle part of the small intestine.

The pancreas

The pancreas is located behind the stomach and next to the spleen. The small intestine wraps around the wide end of the pancreas. The liver and gallbladder are found nearby.

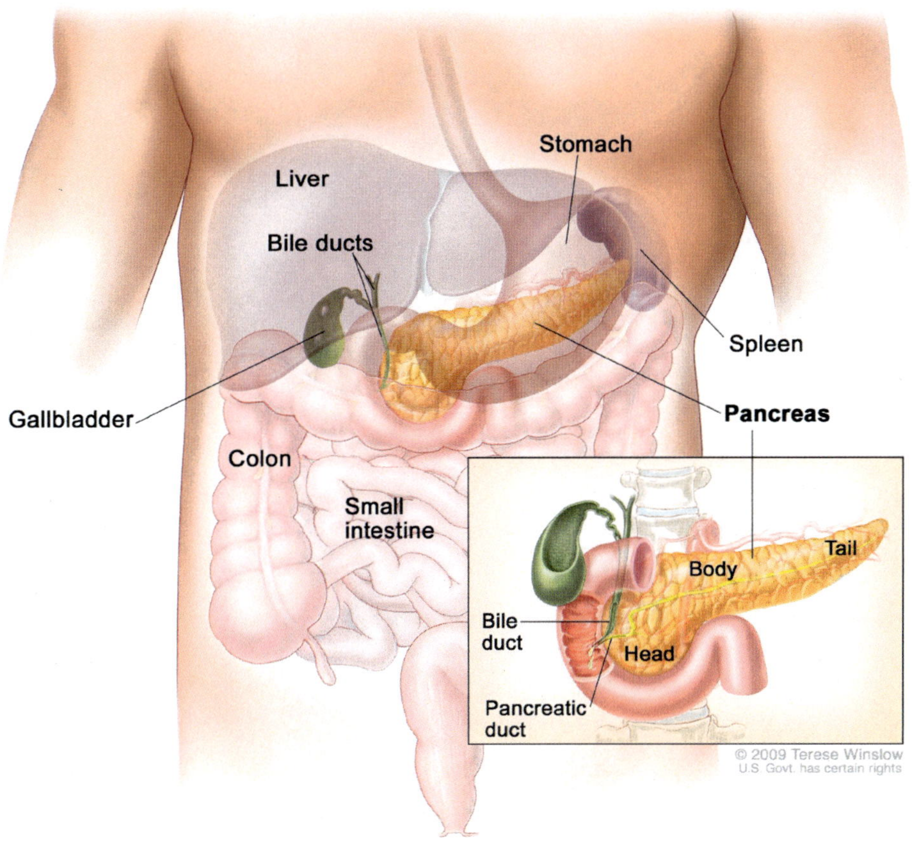

The pancreas has 3 parts:

- Wide end called the head (includes neck and uncinate)
- Middle part called the body
- Narrow end called the tail

The pancreas does 2 important things:

- It makes hormones (insulin and glucagon) that control the amount of sugar (glucose) in your blood. This helps your body use and store energy from food. Removing part of the pancreas might put you at risk for diabetes. If you have diabetes, it might make it worse.
- It makes powerful substances called pancreatic enzymes that helps digest food in your small intestine. Removing part of the pancreas can decrease the amount of these enzymes. This can cause oily diarrhea (watery stool), stools that float, abdominal pain, bloating, gas, and weight loss.

Parts of the pancreas

The pancreas consists of a wide end called the head (includes neck and uncinate process), a middle part called the body, and a narrow end called the tail.

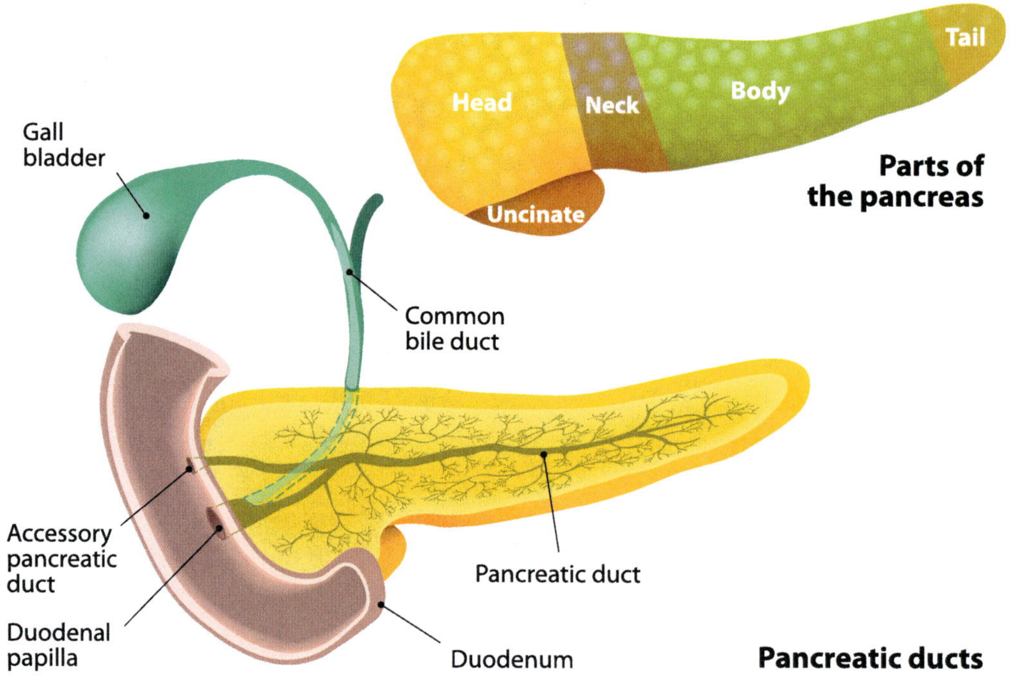

Types of pancreatic cancer

Cancer is a disease that starts in the cells of your body. Most cancers are named after the cell from which they formed. Pancreatic cancer starts in exocrine or endocrine cells of the pancreas. Cancer that forms in the ampulla of Vater (ducts from the liver and pancreas that enter at the small intestine) is often mistaken for pancreatic cancer.

Endocrine

Endocrine cells of the pancreas make hormones. These are released directly into the bloodstream.

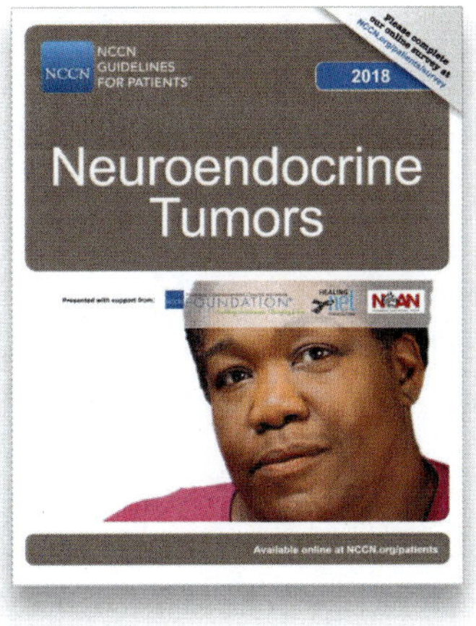

Information on neuroendocrine tumors can be found in *NCCN Guidelines for Patients: Neuroendocrine Tumors*, available at NCCN.org/patientguidelines.

Exocrine

An exocrine cell makes or secretes enzymes into the small intestine that helps digest food. Sometimes, pancreatic cancer is also called exocrine cancer. About 9 out of 10 pancreatic cancers start in exocrine cells that line small tubes called ducts of the pancreas. These ducts carry fluid that contain enzymes into the main pancreatic duct and then into the small intestine. Most pancreatic cancers are ductal adenocarcinomas. An adenocarcinoma is cancer in the cells that secrete fluids or other substances.

Exocrine pancreatic cancer is called pancreatic ductal adenocarcinoma (PDAC) and is the focus of this book. PDAC can grow anywhere in the pancreas, but it is most often found in the head of the pancreas.

Risk factors

Anything that increases your chances of developing cancer is called a risk factor. Risk factors can be activities people do, things you have contact with in the environment, or traits passed down from parents to children through genes. Genes are coded instructions for your cells. Risk factors for pancreatic cancer can be found in Guide 1.

Guide 1
Pancreatic cancer risk factors

Tobacco smoking
Heavy alcohol use
High body mass index (BMI) or excess weight
Genetics
Lack of exercise
Pre-diabetes
Chronic pancreatitis
Long-term diabetes
Long-term use of diabetes medicine
Periodontal disease
Family history of pancreatitis
Family history of pancreatic cancer
Contact with chemicals and heavy metals

Genetic predisposition

Certain genetic changes, or mutations, can increase your chances of developing pancreatic cancer. In a process called mutation something goes wrong in the genetic code. Mutations may have been present in the DNA you inherited from your parents or may be caused later in life by genetic damage (acquired). People with inherited genetic mutations have a higher risk for certain cancers.

A syndrome is a set of symptoms or conditions that occur together and suggest the presence of a certain disease or an increased chance of developing the disease.

Some cancer-related genetic syndromes that increase the risk for pancreatic cancer include:

- Peutz-Jeghers syndrome is caused by mutations in the *STK11* gene.
- Familial pancreatitis is caused by *PRSS1*, *SPINK1*, or *CFTR* gene mutations.
- Lynch syndrome is caused by mutations in mismatch repair (MMR) genes (*MLH1, MSH2, MSH6,* or *PMS2*).
- Hereditary breast-ovarian cancer syndrome is caused by *BRCA1* and/or *BRCA2* mutations.
- Familial malignant melanoma syndrome, also known as melanoma-pancreatic cancer syndrome or familial atypical multiple mole melanoma (FAMMM) syndrome, is caused by mutation of the *CDKN2A* gene.
- Familial pancreatitis is a genetic disorder that runs in families.

Share what you know about your family history with your doctor. This includes if you are of Ashkenazi Jewish ancestry.

Your health care provider might refer you for genetic testing for inherited mutations to learn more about your cancer. A genetic counselor or geneticist will speak to you about the results.

Symptoms

There are no screening tests to detect pancreatic cancer early. It is important to tell your health care provider how you are feeling. If your doctor suspects pancreatic cancer, you will have imaging and other tests.

Seek care with a specialist if you have any of the possible pancreatic cancer symptoms listed in Guide 2.

Guide 2 **Possible pancreatic cancer symptoms**
Weight loss
Darker urine, pale or floating stools
Nausea
Vomiting
Jaundice (yellowing of the skin and eyes)
Indigestion (heartburn, pain, fullness in belly)
Pain in the abdomen or back
Pancreatitis
Trouble controlling diabetes
New-onset diabetes
New-onset blood clots in the veins of the legs (deep vein thrombosis)
New-onset blood clots in the lung (pulmonary embolism)

How cancer spreads

Cancer cells can spread through the blood and lymphatic system and form tumors in other parts of the body. Cancer that has spread is called a metastasis.

- Cancer that has spread to a nearby organ or lymph node is called a local metastasis or locally advanced. In locally advanced pancreatic cancer, cancer has spread to nearby blood vessels and it may be in nearby lymph nodes.
- Cancer that has spread to an area far from the primary tumor is called a distant metastasis. Pancreatic cancer can metastasize in the liver, spleen, stomach, lungs, and other parts of the body.

Cancer can spread to distant sites through blood. Two major blood vessels lie behind the pancreas. The superior mesenteric artery supplies the intestines with blood. The superior mesenteric vein returns blood to the heart. Pancreatic cancer can travel through these blood vessels and metastasize in the liver, spleen, stomach, lungs, and other parts of the body.

Cancer can also spread through the lymphatic system. The lymphatic system has a clear fluid called lymph. Lymph gives cells water and food. It also has white blood cells that fight germs. Lymph nodes filter lymph and remove the germs. Lymph travels throughout the body in vessels like blood does. Lymph vessels and nodes are found everywhere in the body.

Review

- The pancreas makes hormones, such as insulin. It also makes proteins, called enzymes, which help to digest food.
- Pancreatic cancer often starts in the exocrine cells that line the ducts of the pancreas.
- There are no screening tests to detect pancreatic cancer early.
- Anything that increases your chances of cancer is called a risk factor.
- Genetic mutations inherited from your parents can increase your chance of developing pancreatic and other cancers.
- Cancer cells can spread to other areas of the body through blood or lymph.

2
Testing for pancreatic cancer

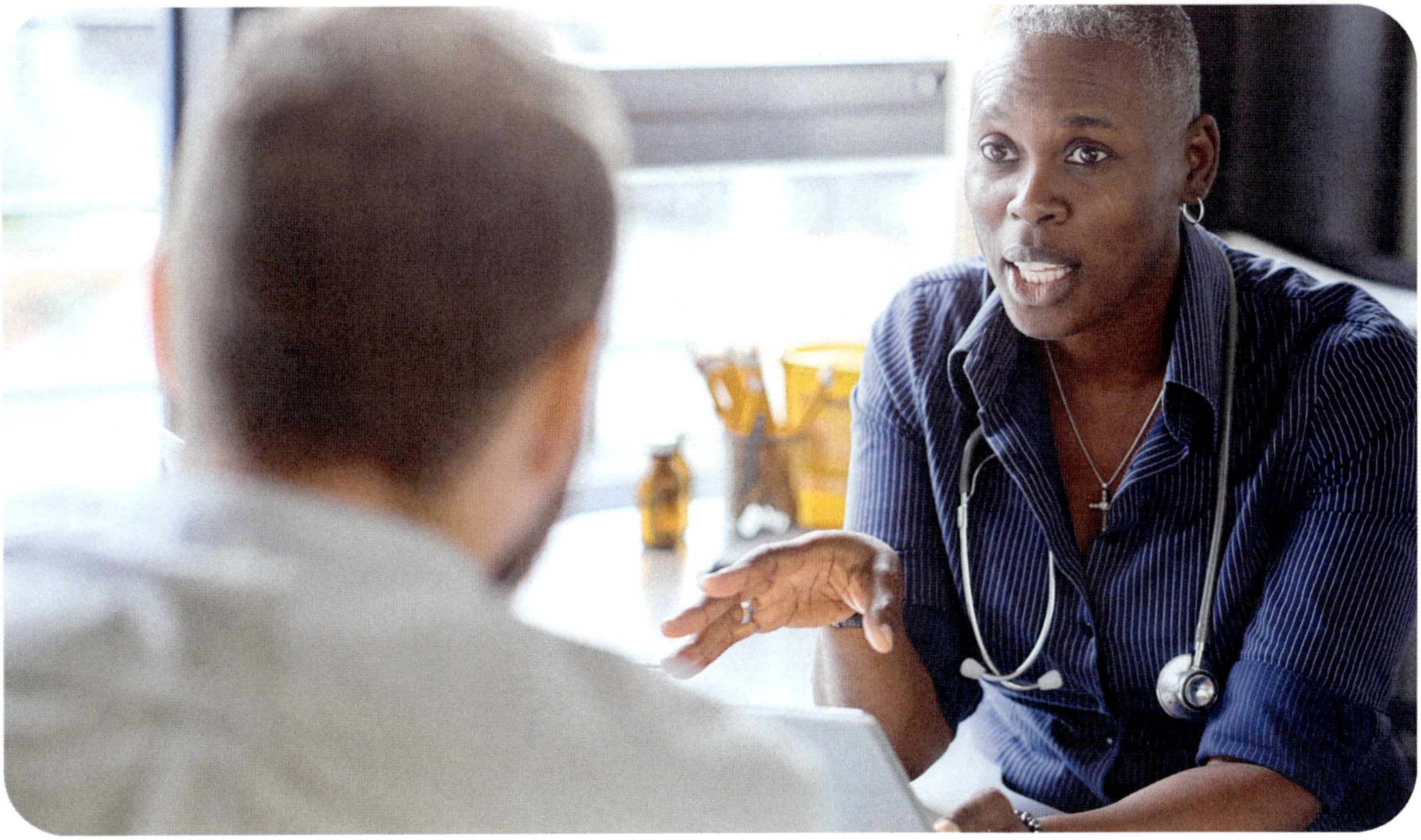

Treatment planning starts with testing. Imaging is used to confirm pancreatic cancer. This chapter outlines tests used in the diagnosis and treatment of pancreatic cancer.

Test results

Results from imaging studies, blood tests, and biopsies will determine your treatment plan. It is important you understand what these tests mean. Ask questions and keep copies of your test results. Online patient portals are a great way to access your test results.

Keep these things in mind:

- Bring someone with you to doctor visits, if possible.
- Write down questions and take notes during appointments. Don't be afraid to ask your care team questions. Get to know your care team and let them get to know you.
- Get copies of blood tests, imaging results, and reports about the specific type of cancer you have. It will be helpful when getting a second opinion.
- Organize your papers. Create files for insurance forms, medical records, and test results. You can do the same on your computer.
- Keep a list of contact information for everyone on your care team. Add it to your phone. Hang the list on your fridge or keep it in a place where someone can access it in an emergency.

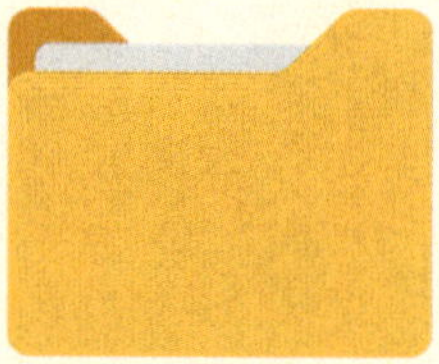

Create a medical binder

A medical binder or notebook is a great way to organize all of your records in one place.

- Make copies of blood tests, imaging results, and reports about your specific type of cancer.
- Choose a binder that meets your needs. Consider a zipper pocket to include a pen, small calendar, and insurance cards.
- Create folders for insurance forms, medical records, and tests results. You can do the same on your computer.
- Use online patient portals to view your test results and other records. Download or print the records to add to your binder.
- Organize your binder in a way that works for you. Add a section for questions and to take notes.
- Bring your medical binder to appointments. You never know when you might need it!

General health tests

Medical history

A medical history is a record of all health issues and treatments you have had in your life. Be prepared to list any illness or injury and when it happened. Bring a list of old and new medicines and any over-the-counter medicines, herbals, or supplements you take. Tell your doctor about any symptoms you have. A medical history will help determine which treatment is best for you.

Family history

Some cancers and other diseases can run in families. Your doctor will ask about the health history of family members who are blood relatives. This information is called a family history. It is important to ask members from both parents' side of the family about all cancers, not just pancreatic cancer. Ask about other health issues like heart disease and diabetes, at what age they were diagnosed, and if anyone died from their cancer. Share this information and any changes to family history with your health care provider.

Physical exam

During a physical exam, your health care provider may:

- Check your temperature, blood pressure, pulse, and breathing rate
- Check your weight
- Listen to your lungs and heart
- Look in your eyes, ears, nose, and throat
- Feel and apply pressure to parts of your body to see if organs are of normal size, are soft or hard, or cause pain when touched. Tell your doctor if you feel pain.
- Feel for enlarged lymph nodes in your neck, underarm, and groin. Tell the doctor if you have felt any lumps or have any pain.
- Check for signs of jaundice, a yellowing of the skin and eyes

Jaundice is caused by a buildup of bilirubin in the body. Bilirubin is a yellow-brown substance found in bile. Bilirubin forms when red blood cells are broken down in bile. Bile is a chemical made by the liver that helps digest fat. Bile flows through bile ducts in the liver into the intestines. A tumor in the pancreas can cause jaundice by blocking the main bile duct. When that happens, your bowel movements may turn pale, yellow-orange in color, and your urine becomes darker. Severe jaundice can cause itchy skin, as well.

Blood tests

Blood tests check for signs of disease and how well organs are working. They require a sample of your blood, which is removed through a needle placed into your vein.

Liver function tests

Liver function tests look at the health of your liver by measuring chemicals that are made or processed by the liver. Levels that are too high or low signal that the liver is not working well or the bile ducts might be blocked.

Bilirubin levels will be measured. Bilirubin is a chemical that gives bile its color. Bilirubin forms when red blood cells are broken down in bile. There may be too much bilirubin in the blood if a tumor is blocking a bile duct and preventing the free flow of bile from the liver into the intestines. Too much bilirubin causes a yellowing of the eyes and skin called jaundice and dark-colored urine.

CA 19-9

Carbohydrate antigen (CA) 19-9 is a substance found in blood that is often high in people with pancreatic cancer. This test is not used by itself to diagnose pancreatic cancer. Other health problems besides pancreatic cancer can cause high levels of CA 19-9.

Imaging tests

Imaging tests take pictures of the inside of your body. A radiologist, an expert in interpreting imaging tests, will write a report and send this report to your doctor. Your doctor will discuss the results with you.

There is more than one type of imaging test that may be used for pancreatic cancer. Images can be made with scanning machines or scoping tools. The images may show if there is a tumor in your pancreas as well as the tumor size and location. You will have imaging tests at diagnosis and throughout your treatment to see how the cancer is responding.

The types of imaging tests recommended for pancreatic cancer are described next.

CT scan

A computed tomography (CT or CAT) scan uses x-rays and computer technology to take pictures of the inside of the body. It takes many x-rays of the same body part from different angles. All the images are combined to make one detailed picture. In most cases, contrast given by vein injection will be used. Contrast materials are not dyes, but substances that help enhance and improve the images of several organs and structures in the body. It is used to make the pictures clearer. The contrast is not permanent and will leave the body in your urine immediately after the test.

Tell your doctors if you have had allergic reactions to contrast in the past. This is important. You might be given medicines, such as Benadryl® and prednisone, to avoid the effects of those allergies. Contrast might not be used if you have a serious allergy or if your kidneys aren't working well.

Pancreatic protocol CT scan

A special type of CT scan, called a pancreatic protocol CT scan, is recommended for those with pancreatic cancer. A protocol is a detailed plan of a medical study, treatment, or procedure. A pancreatic protocol CT is adjusted for the best view of the pancreas and nearby organs. This allows doctors to clearly see where the tumor is in the pancreas and if the tumor involves any veins, arteries, or organs. A pancreatic protocol CT will also help to see if there are metastases outside the pancreas.

When your doctor suspects pancreatic cancer or that there might be an issue with your pancreatic or bile ducts, a pancreatic protocol CT is usually the first test.

MRI scan

A magnetic resonance imaging (MRI) scan uses radio waves and powerful magnets to take pictures of the inside of the body. It does not use x-rays. An MRI may cause your body to feel a bit warm. Like a CT scan, a contrast material injected into a vein is often used to make the pictures clearer. An MRI is only done in certain cases. It is commonly used to look for liver metastases or to evaluate small tumors in the pancreas.

Pancreatic protocol MRI scan

A special type of MRI scan, called a pancreatic protocol MRI scan, is recommended for pancreatic cancer. A pancreatic protocol MRI scan is adjusted for the best view of the pancreas and nearby organs. This special MRI scan allows doctors to clearly see the pancreas, nearby blood vessels, and very small tumors. For some people, a pancreatic protocol MRI scan may be used instead of CT to view the pancreas.

MRCP

A magnetic resonance cholangiopancreatography (MRCP) is a type of MRI scan that makes very clear pictures of the pancreas and bile ducts. No contrast is used because bile and other fluids act as their own contrast. An MRCP is usually done with an MRI scan.

PET scan

A positron emission tomography (PET) scan uses a radioactive drug called a tracer. A tracer is a substance injected into a vein to see where cancer cells are in the body and if they are using sugar to grow. Cancer cells show up as bright spots on PET scans. Not all bright spots are cancer. It is normal for the brain, heart, kidneys, and bladder to be bright on PET. When a PET scan is combined with CT, it is called a PET/CT scan. A PET scan is only done in certain cases.

Scoping tests

Some imaging tests use a thin, tube-shaped tool called a scope that is inserted into the body to take pictures. One end of the scope has a small light and camera lens to see inside your body. The image is sent to a television monitor. This will guide your doctor in a biopsy, stent placement, or other tasks.

The scope is guided into the body through a natural opening, such as the mouth or nose. It may also be inserted through a small surgical cut.

More than one type of scope may be used for imaging tests. The type of scope often used for pancreatic cancer is called an endoscope. An endoscope is often guided into the body through the mouth.

There are 3 types of imaging tests with scopes used for pancreatic cancer:

- Endoscopic ultrasound (EUS)
- Endoscopic retrograde cholangiopancreatography (ERCP)
- Laparoscopy

Endoscope

An endoscope is a thin tube-shaped tool with a camera. It is inserted through your mouth and used to look inside your body.

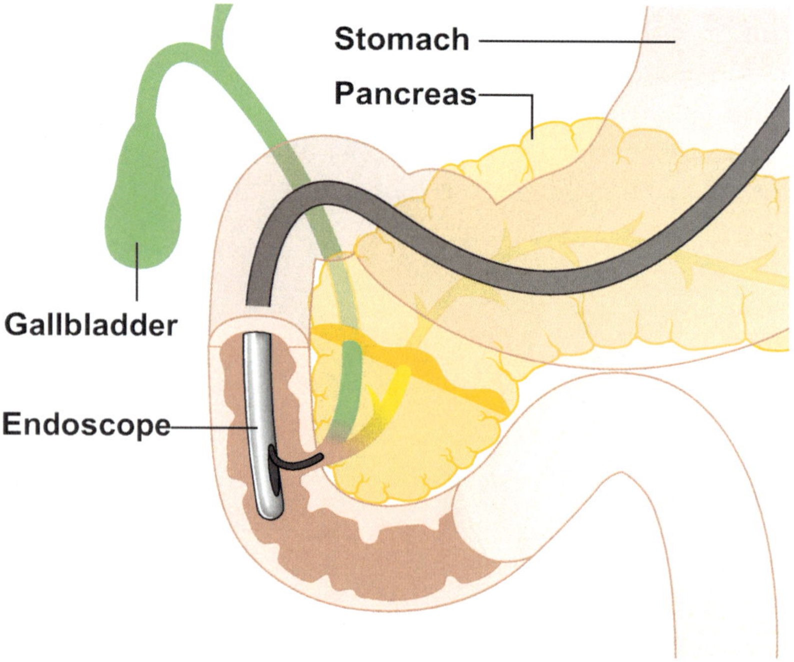

EUS

An EUS uses an endoscope that has a small ultrasound probe at the end. The endoscope is inserted through your mouth and guided down your throat and stomach to the first part of the small intestine (duodenum). The ultrasound probe bounces sound waves off your pancreas and other organs to make pictures of the inside of your body.

EUS is used to guide a biopsy of your pancreas and to stage a tumor. Sometimes an EUS can detect small lesions in the pancreas that are difficult to see on a CT or MRI scan.

An EUS is done under sedation to keep you comfortable during the procedure. It might be done with an ERCP.

ERCP

An ERCP uses an endoscope and x-rays to make moving pictures of the inside of the body. For this test, the endoscope will be inserted through your mouth and guided down your throat and stomach to the duodenum. Next, a thinner tube called a catheter will be passed through the middle of the endoscope. The catheter will be used to inject a contrast material into the pancreatic and bile ducts. The contrast material allows the ducts to be clearly seen on the x-ray pictures.

A tumor can cause a blocked bile duct. An ERCP is used to open a blocked bile duct by allowing placing a plastic or metal stent to keep the bile duct open. During an ERCP, biopsy samples may be taken from the common bile duct. Samples are removed with a small brush at the end of the endoscope. These samples are called brushings. Brushings are taken before stent placement.

An ERCP is done under sedation to keep you comfortable during the procedure. It might be done with an EUS.

Laparoscopy

This test is a type of surgery that allows your doctors to see organs in your abdomen. It uses a tool like an endoscope called a laparoscope to look for metastases. For this test, the laparoscope will be inserted through a tiny cut in your abdomen. Laparoscopy is done under general anesthesia. This is a controlled loss of wakefulness from drugs. A pancreatic tumor might be biopsied during surgery or laparoscopy.

Biopsy

A biopsy is the removal of a tissue or group of cells for testing. To confirm pancreatic cancer, you will have a biopsy. The biopsy might be done during another procedure, during surgery to remove the tumor, or by itself. Tests will be done on the biopsied cells.

A pathologist is an expert who will test the biopsy for cancer and write a report called a pathology report. The pathologist may perform other tests to see if the cancer cells have specific genes or proteins. This information will help choose the best treatment plan for your type of cancer. Ask questions about your biopsy results and what it means for your cancer treatment.

If no cancer cells are found, a biopsy may be taken from another part of the pancreas. Biopsies are usually the final step in a cancer diagnosis. You might need more than one biopsy and more than one type of biopsy. Ask your health care provider about the type of biopsy you will have and what you can do to get ready.

The different types of biopsies are described next.

Brushings

Brushings are tumor or cell samples removed with a small brush at the end of the endoscope, usually during an ERCP procedure.

FNA

A fine-needle aspiration (FNA) biopsy uses a very thin needle to remove the tissue sample. It is the most common type of biopsy used to confirm pancreatic cancer. FNA biopsies can be done through EUS or guided by a CT or ultrasound.

EUS-FNA

An EUS-guided FNA biopsy or EUS-FNA uses a thin needle attached to the end of the endoscope. An endoscope uses a lighted scope passed through the mouth and throat down into your stomach. An ultrasound probe at the end of the endoscope bounces sound waves off organs and tissues to make a picture of the inside of your body. Your doctor uses these pictures to guide the endoscope and needle to the right spot. Then the needle is inserted through your stomach or duodenum and into the tumor in your pancreas to remove a tissue sample. If cancer is confined to the pancreas, an EUS-guided biopsy is preferred to prevent tumor spreading. You might have more than one EUS-guided biopsy.

CT or ultrasound-guided FNA

In a CT or ultrasound-guided FNA biopsy, a thin needle is inserted through the skin and into the tumor using a CT scan or ultrasound as a guide to find the right spot. The CT scan takes many pictures of a part of the body from different angles using x-rays. An ultrasound is a test that uses sound waves to take pictures of the inside of the body. Your doctor will use these pictures to find the tumor in your pancreas and guide the needle to the right spot. For this type of biopsy, you will be given local anesthesia. It is called local because this anesthesia causes a loss of feeling in a small area of the body.

Genetic testing

Genetic (germline) testing is recommended for anyone with confirmed pancreatic cancer. Germline testing is done using blood or saliva (spitting into a cup). The goal is to look for gene mutations inherited from your parents called germline mutations. Some mutations can put you at risk for more than one type of cancer. You can pass these genes on to your children. Also, family members might carry these mutations. Tell your doctor if there is a family history of cancer, especially pancreatic cancer.

Some types of germline mutations for pancreatic cancer include:

- *BRCA1*
- *BRCA2*
- *PALB2*

If you have one or more of these germline mutations, your doctor might choose a platinum-based systemic therapy or a treatment that is known to work better for your mutation. You might notice that some of the germline mutations like *BRCA1, BRCA2,* or *PALB2* are related to other cancers such as breast, ovarian, prostate, colorectal, or melanoma skin cancer.

Tell your doctor if there is a family history of cancer, especially pancreatic cancer.

Biomarker testing

A tissue sample from the biopsy of your tumor will be tested to look for biomarkers or proteins. Tumor testing is recommended for those with locally advanced or metastatic disease. It is sometimes called gene profiling or molecular testing.

Biomarker testing includes tests of genes or their products (proteins). It identifies the presence or absence of mutations and certain proteins that might affect treatment. Proteins are written like this: BRCA. Genes are written like this: *BRCA.*

Immunohistochemistry (IHC), polymerase chain reaction (PCR), or next-generation sequencing (NGS) are types of tests that will be used to detect the following:

- Some gene fusions include: *ALK, NRG1, NTRK,* and *ROS1*
- Some gene mutations include: *BRAF, BRCA1, BRCA2, HER2, KRAS, PALB2,* and mismatch repair (MMR)

Immunohistochemistry

Immunohistochemistry (IHC) is a special staining process that involves adding a chemical marker to immune cells. The cells are then studied using a microscope.

MSI-H/dMMR mutation

Microsatellites are short, repeated strings of DNA. When errors or defects occur, they are fixed by mismatch repair (MMR) genes. Some cancers prevent these errors from being fixed. This is called microsatellite instability (MSI) or deficient mismatch repair (dMMR). When cancer cells have more than a normal number of microsatellites, it is called MSI-H (microsatellite instability-high). This is often due to deficient MMR genes.

Next-generation sequencing

Next-generation sequencing (NGS) is a high-throughput method used to determine a portion of a person's DNA sequence.

PCR

A polymerase chain reaction (PCR) is a lab process that can make millions or billions of copies of your DNA (genetic information). PCR is very sensitive. It can find 1 abnormal cell among more than 100,000 normal cells. These copies called PCR product might be used for NGS.

Review

- Tests are used to plan treatment and check how well treatment is working.
- In pancreatic cancer, staging is first done using imaging tests.
- A biopsy is needed to confirm pancreatic cancer.
- It is important to know as much as you can about your cancer. Genetic (germline) and biomarker (tumor) testing may give your doctors more information about your cancer, and possible treatment options.

3

Pancreatic cancer treatment

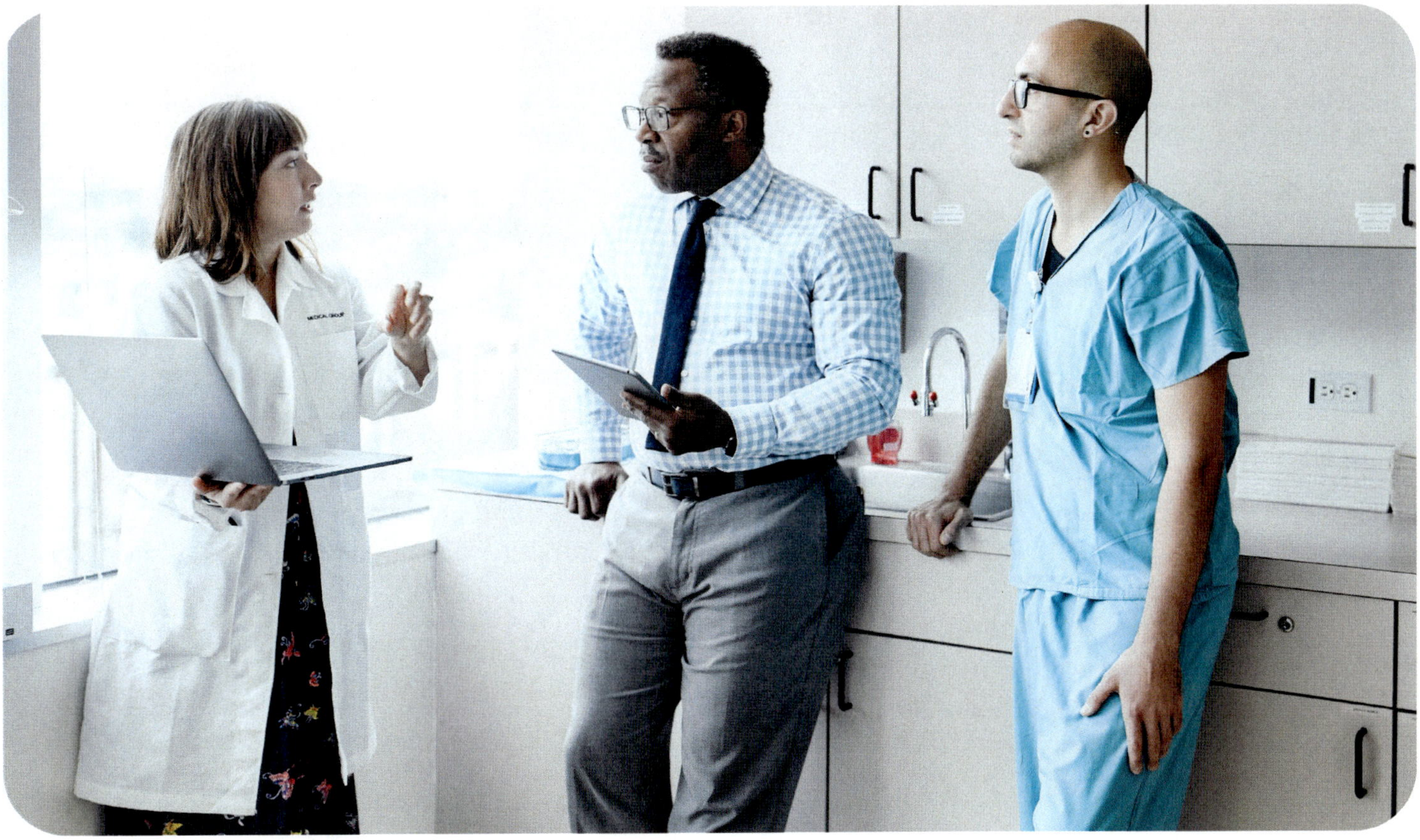

Treatment is based on staging. Staging is done using imaging tests. This chapter presents an overview of the types of treatment and what to expect. Not everyone will receive the same treatment. Together, you and your doctor will choose a treatment plan that is right for you.

Multidisciplinary team

Those with pancreatic cancer should seek treatment at experienced cancer centers.

Treating pancreatic cancer takes a team approach. Treatment decisions should involve a multidisciplinary team (MDT). An MDT is a team of doctors, health care workers, and social care professionals from different professional backgrounds who have knowledge (expertise) and experience with your type of cancer. This team is united in the planning and implementing of your treatment. Ask who will coordinate your care.

Depending on your cancer stage, the team might include:

- **A gastroenterologist** is an expert in diseases of the digestive system and an expert in endoscopic procedures for diagnostic, therapeutic, or palliative purposes.
- **A medical oncologist** treats cancer in adults using systemic therapy. Often, this person will lead the overall treatment team and keep track of tests and exams done by other specialists.
- **Oncology nurses** provide your hands-on care, like giving systemic therapy, managing your care, answering questions, and helping you cope with side effects.
- **Palliative care nurses and advanced practice providers** help provide an extra layer of support with your cancer-related symptoms.
- **An anesthesiologist** gives anesthesia, a medicine so you do not feel pain during surgery or procedures.
- **A diagnostic radiologist** interprets the results of x-rays and other imaging tests.
- **A dietitian or nutritionist** provides guidance on what foods or diet are most suitable for your condition.
- **A pathologist** studies the cells, tissues, and organs removed during a biopsy or surgery.
- **A genetic counselor** assesses your risk for having an inherited type of cancer, and performs germline genetic testing.
- **A radiation oncologist** prescribes and plans radiation therapy to treat cancer and provide palliative care.
- **A surgical oncologist** performs operations to remove cancer.
- **Psychologists and psychiatrists** are mental health experts who can help manage issues such as depression, anxiety, or other mental health conditions that can affect how you feel.
- **Social workers** help people solve and cope with problems in their everyday lives.

Some members of your care team will be with you throughout cancer treatment, while others will only be there for parts of it. Get to know your care team and let them get to know you.

Keep a list of names and contact information for each member of your team. This will make it easier for you and anyone involved in your care to know whom to contact with questions or concerns.

You know your body better than anyone. Help other team members understand:

- How you feel
- What you need
- What is working and what is not
- Your goals for treatment

Cancer is suspected

If pancreatic cancer is suspected, then you will have pancreatic protocol CT of the abdomen. Other possible tests can be found in Guide 3.

A multidisciplinary team of doctors will discuss your test results and agree on the best way to treat your cancer. Multidisciplinary review should ideally involve expertise from diagnostic imaging, interventional endoscopy, medical oncology, radiation oncology, surgery, pathology, and palliative care.

Cancer that has spread to tissues that line and cover the organs in your abdomen are hard to see with imaging tests. Sometimes, cancer cells are too small to be seen. These cells can grow into cancer later. A staging laparoscopy can look for metastases not found on imaging tests.

Guide 3 Possible tests and procedures
Chest and pelvic CT
Endoscopic ultrasonography (EUS)
MRI of lesions
PET/CT
Endoscopic retrograde cholangiopancreatography (ERCP) with stent placement
Liver function test and baseline CA 19-9 after adequate biliary drainage
Genetic (germline) testing if diagnosis confirmed

Metastatic disease

If metastatic disease is suspected, then a biopsy is needed to confirm metastatic disease. It is preferred that a metastasis be biopsied. This will be followed by germline testing, gene profiling of tumor tissue, and complete staging with chest and pelvic CT.

Staging

A cancer stage is a way to describe the extent of the cancer based on test results at the time you are first diagnosed with cancer. Staging is needed to plan and monitor treatment. In pancreatic cancer, imaging tests are used to stage cancer. This is different than other cancers.

Staging starts with a pancreatic protocol CT and other imaging tests. These tests determine if the tumor can be removed with surgery (resectable), if the disease has spread to nearby organs or lymph nodes (locally advanced), or if it has spread to distant areas of the body (metastasized). See Guide 4.

Guide 4
Pancreatic cancer groups based on before-surgery imaging tests

	What does it mean?	Can surgery be done?	Why?
Resectable	Cancer has not spread outside the pancreas.	Yes, tumor can be removed completely with surgery.	Tumor has not grown into nearby arteries or veins.
Borderline resectable	It is hard to tell from imaging tests if the cancer has spread to nearby tissues.	It is unclear if the tumor can be removed with surgery.	Tumor may or may not have grown into nearby arteries and veins.
Locally advanced	There is cancer (metastasis) in nearby lymph nodes and tissues.	Tumor and nearby lymph nodes may or may not be removed with surgery.	Tumor has grown or may involve major blood vessels that cannot be removed or reconstructed.
Metastatic	Cancer has spread to distant parts of the body.	No, tumor cannot be removed with surgery.	Tumor has grown into surrounding tissues and has spread to distant parts of the body.

This book will use the following terms to stage or describe pancreatic cancer:

- **Resectable –** Tumor can be removed completely with surgery.
- **Borderline resectable –** Sometimes, imaging tests cannot clearly show one way or the other if surgery is an option. In borderline resectable pancreatic cancer, the tumor involves nearby veins and arteries.
- **Locally advanced –** Cancer that has spread to nearby lymph nodes, organs, and tissues. Lymph nodes can be found along the ducts, veins, and arteries of the pancreas, liver, spleen, and other organs.
- **Metastatic –** Cancer that has spread to other parts of the body, including distant lymph nodes. The most common metastatic sites are the liver, abdomen, lungs, and bone.

Performance status

Performance status (PS) is a person's general level of fitness. Your state of general health will be rated using a PS scale called ECOG (Eastern Cooperative Oncology Group). PS scale scores or grades range from 0 to 4. This score helps doctors decide what kind of pancreatic cancer treatment is best for you.

- PS 0 means you are fully active.
- PS 1 means you are still able to perform light to moderate activity.
- PS 2 means you can still care for yourself but are not active.
- PS 3 means you are limited to the chair or bed more than half of the time.
- PS 4 means you need someone to care for you and are limited to a chair or bed.

In pancreatic cancer treatment, PS will be referred to as good or poor. Good PS is usually PS 0 or PS 1.

Surgery

Surgery is an operation or procedure to remove cancer from the body. Sometimes, surgery can be used as the main or primary treatment to remove the cancer from the pancreas. This is only one part of a treatment plan. Surgery can also provide supportive care by easing pain or discomfort.

Surgery for pancreatic cancer should be done at a center that does at least 15 to 20 pancreatic surgeries each year. Hospitals that perform many pancreatic surgeries often have better results.

The type of surgery you receive depends on size and location of the tumor in the pancreas. It also depends on if there is cancer in any surrounding organs and tissues.

There are 2 types of surgery:

- Open surgery
- Minimally invasive surgery (laparoscopic or robotic surgery)

Open surgery

Open surgery or laparotomy removes tissue through one large surgical cut below your ribs. The large cut lets your doctor directly view and access the tumor in your pancreas to remove it. Open surgery may take several hours or longer. After the surgery, you will need to stay in the hospital for several days or longer to recover.

Minimally invasive surgery

Minimally invasive surgery uses a few small incisions or cuts instead of one large one. Small tools are inserted through each incision to perform the surgery. One of the tools, called a laparoscope, is a long tube with a video camera at the end. The camera lets your doctor see your pancreas and other tissues inside your abdomen. Other tools are used to remove the tumor. Laparoscopic surgery can also be done using robotic arms to control the surgical tools. This is called robot-assisted laparoscopic surgery.

Tumor resection

Imaging tests will be ordered to see if your cancer is resectable (can be removed completely by surgery) or unresectable (cannot be removed completely by surgery). Sometimes, imaging tests cannot clearly show one way or the other. In this case, pancreatic cancer is called borderline resectable. In borderline resectable pancreatic cancer, the tumor involves nearby veins and arteries.

Goal of surgery

The goal of surgery or tumor resection is to remove all the cancer. To do so, the tumor is removed along with some normal-looking tissue around its edge. The normal-looking tissue is called the surgical margin. A clear or negative margin (R0) is when no cancer cells are found in the tissue around the edge of the tumor. In a positive margin cancer cells are found in normal-looking tissue around the tumor. R0 resection is very difficult to achieve in pancreatic cancer. Even with an R0 resection, the chance of cancer returning (recurrence) is high.

A negative margin (R0) is the best result. Your surgeon will look carefully for cancer not only along the surgical margin, but in other nearby areas. If your doctor does not feel a negative margin is possible, you may not be able to have the cancer removed right away. Instead the surgeon may recommend for you to receive a systemic treatment before surgery called neoadjuvant therapy. Neoadjuvant therapy will help shrink the size of the tumor and the amount of cancer in the body.

Types of pancreatic surgery

There are 3 types of surgery to remove tumors in the pancreas.

- **Pancreaticoduodenectomy –** Surgery that removes the head of the pancreas, gallbladder, duodenum (first part of the small intestine), part of the bile duct, nearby lymph nodes, and often part of the stomach. This is known as a Whipple procedure. This surgery can be open or minimally invasive.
- **Distal pancreatectomy –** Surgery that removes the body and tail of the pancreas, and sometimes the entire spleen (splenectomy). The left adrenal gland might also be removed. This surgery can be open or minimally invasive.
- **Total pancreatectomy –** Surgery that removes the whole pancreas, part of the small intestine, part of the stomach, the common bile duct, the gallbladder, the spleen, and nearby lymph nodes. It is usually done as open surgery.

Your team will gather as much information as possible before surgery. Often, it is very hard to know until surgery how much cancer there is and if the cancer involves any veins, arteries, lymph nodes, and other organs. Complex decisions must be made during surgery. Ask your surgeon what might be removed during surgery and what this means. Sometimes, a tumor will be found to be unresectable during surgery. At this time, a biopsy will be done if one was not done before. A biopsy will help with treatment options.

Whipple procedure

If the tumor is in the head of your pancreas, you will have a pancreaticoduodenectomy (Whipple procedure). A Whipple procedure is surgery that removes the head of the pancreas, the gallbladder, duodenum (first part of the small intestine), part of the bile duct, and often part of the stomach.

Lymph nodes near your pancreas will be removed and tested. Once the cancer has been removed, your surgeons will reconnect your organs so you can digest food. Possible life-threatening complications of this surgery are infection, bleeding, pancreatic leaks, and fistulas (an opening between organs).

A Whipple procedure can be open or minimally invasive. It requires a great deal of skill. Blood vessels might have to be removed or pieces cut out and sewn back together. Parts of organs might have to be removed and sewn back together. All cancer must be removed to achieve a negative margin resection (R0). This might not be possible based on the type and stage of pancreatic cancer.

Whipple procedure

The image on the left shows cancer in the head of the pancreas. The image on the right shows how the organs might be reconnected during a Whipple procedure.

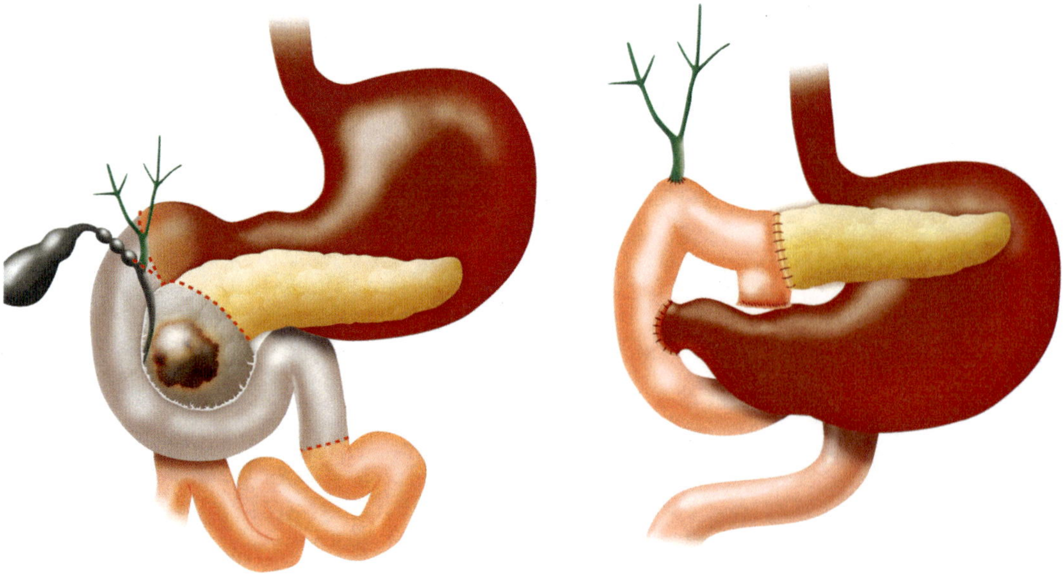

Distal pancreatectomy

A distal pancreatectomy is a surgery to remove the body and tail of the pancreas. It is possible the entire spleen will have to be removed (splenectomy) if there is cancer in the spleen or its vessels. Two out of 5 people have their spleen removed with a distal pancreatectomy. Other blood vessels might have to be removed or pieces cut out and sewn back together. The left adrenal gland might be removed. Cancer in this area of the pancreas is usually more advanced. Even with R0 resection, local recurrence is possible.

Total pancreatectomy

A total pancreatectomy removes the whole pancreas, part of the small intestine, part of the stomach, the common bile duct, the gallbladder, nearby lymph nodes, and the spleen (splenectomy). This surgery is rare. It is done when there are multiple tumors or when there is cancer throughout the pancreas.

Surgical bed

When part or all of the pancreas has been removed, the area that remains is called the surgical or operative bed. Cancer may return to this area. This is called a local recurrence and is treated differently than cancer that has returned to the pancreas or cancer that has spread (metastasized) to distant sites in the body.

Surgery

✓ Pancreatic resections should be done at hospitals that perform at least 15 to 20 each year. This is known as a high-volume center.

Pancreatic surgery takes a great deal of skill. Hospitals that perform many pancreatic surgeries often have better results.

Gastrojejunostomy

A gastrojejunostomy is a surgery to re-route the path food takes from the stomach into the small intestine. The new path from the stomach will avoid (bypass) the blocked part of the duodenum. A gastrojejunostomy can be an open surgery or laparoscopic. This surgery may also be done as a preventive measure if there is a high risk that your stomach may become blocked.

J-tube

A jejunostomy tube (J-tube) is a soft, plastic tube placed through the skin of the abdomen into the midsection of the small intestine. The tube delivers food and medicine until you are healthy enough to eat by mouth. A J-tube is possible with a gastrojejunostomy. You will learn how to care for the J-tube and the skin where the tube enters the body.

Digestive system

Cancer can block the stomach or small intestine. Surgery that re-routes the path food takes from the stomach to small intestine is called a gastrojejunostomy.

Digestive Tract

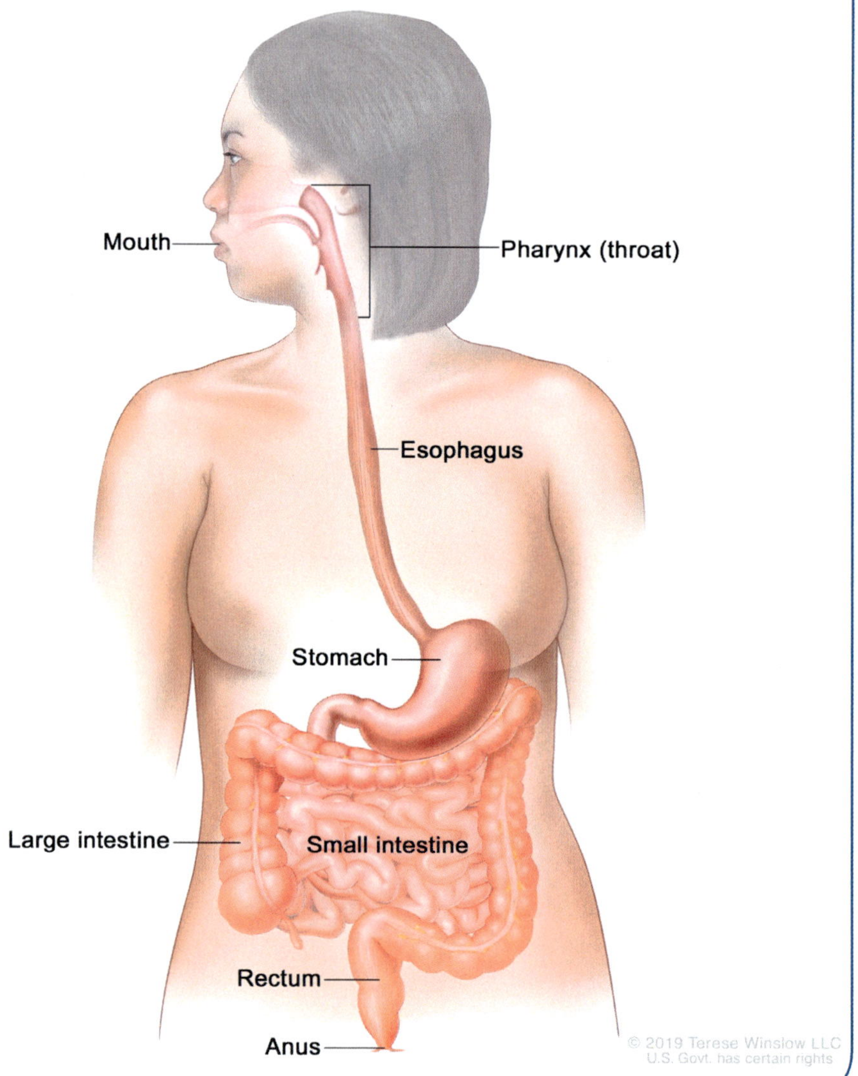

Systemic therapy

Systemic therapy is used in all stages of pancreatic cancer. Systemic therapy works throughout the body. Types include chemotherapy, targeted therapy, and immunotherapy. Systemic therapy might be used alone or with other therapies.

Goals of systemic therapy should be discussed before starting treatment. Your wishes about treatment are important.

- When systemic therapy is given before surgery it is called neoadjuvant therapy.
- When systemic therapy is given after surgery, it is called adjuvant therapy.

Chemotherapy

Chemotherapy kills fast-growing cells throughout the body, including cancer cells and some normal cells. All chemotherapies affect the instructions (genes) that tell cancer cells how and when to grow and divide. There are many chemotherapies used to treat pancreatic cancer. Often chemotherapies are combined. This is called multiagent chemotherapy.

- In gemcitabine-based therapy, gemcitabine is used in combination with other systemic therapies.
- In fluoropyrimidine-based therapy, 5-fluorouracil (5-FU) is used in combination with other systemic therapies.

Did you know?

The terms “chemotherapy” and “systemic therapy” are often used interchangeably, but they are not the same. Chemotherapy, targeted therapy, and immunotherapy are all types of systemic therapy.

Targeted therapy

Targeted therapy focuses on specific or unique features of cancer cells. Targeted therapies seek out how cancer cells grow, divide, and move in the body. These drugs stop the action of molecules that help cancer cells grow and/or survive.

Neurotrophin receptor kinase *(NTRK)* gene fusions are rare in pancreatic cancer. In a tumor with an *NTRK* gene fusion, a piece of the *NTRK* gene and a piece of another gene fuse, or join. This activates the *NTRK* gene in a way that causes uncontrolled cell growth. Larotrectinib and entrectinib are targeted therapies that might be used to target advanced or metastatic cancer that is *NTRK* gene fusion-positive. There are targeted therapies used in clinical trials, which target other genetic mutations or alterations such as *HER2*, *BRAF*, and others.

Immunotherapy

Immunotherapy is a targeted therapy that increases the activity of your own immune system. By doing so, it improves your body's ability to find and destroy cancer cells. Immunotherapy can be given alone or with other types of treatment.

Pembrolizumab is an example of an immunotherapy that targets (blocks) PD-L1 and PD-L2. It might be used for advanced pancreatic cancer for MSI-H or dMMR tumors.

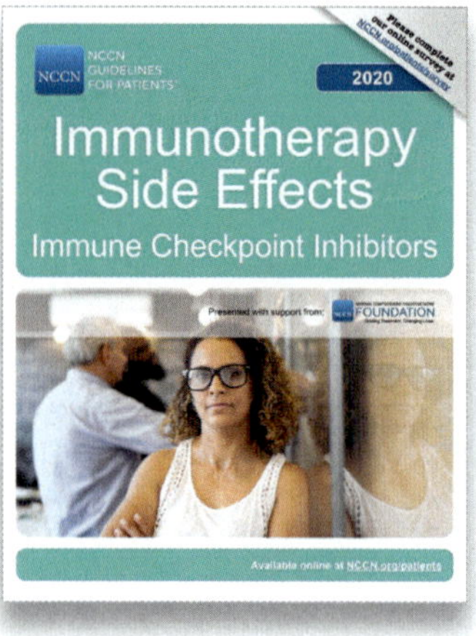

For more information, read the *NCCN Guidelines for Patients: Immunotherapy Side Effects,* available at NCCN.org/patientguidelines.

Tell your doctor about any medicines, vitamins, over-the-counter drugs, herbals, or supplements you are taking.

Warnings!

You might be asked to stop taking or avoid certain herbal supplements when on a systemic therapy. Some supplements can affect the ability of a drug to do its job. This is called a drug interaction. It is critical to speak with your care team about any supplements you may be taking.

Some examples include:

- Turmeric
- Gingko biloba
- Green tea extract
- St. John's Wort

Certain medicines can also affect the ability of a drug to do its job. Antacids, heart medicine, and antidepressants are just some of the medicines that might interact with a systemic therapy. This is why it is important to tell your doctor about any medications, vitamins, over-the-counter (OTC) drugs, herbals, or supplements you are taking. **Bring a list with you to every visit.**

Radiation therapy

Radiation therapy (RT) uses high-energy radiation from x-rays, photons, electrons, and other sources to kill cancer cells and shrink tumors. RT can be given alone or with other treatments. Treatment may focus on individual tumors, a small area/region of the body, or specific lymph nodes. RT may be used as supportive care or palliative care to help ease pain or discomfort caused by cancer.

Radiation therapy can also be given before, during, or after surgery to treat or slow the growth of cancer, especially if the surgical margins have cancer cells.

EBRT

External beam radiation therapy (EBRT) uses a machine outside of the body to aim radiation at the tumor(s) or areas of the body.

Common types of EBRT that may be used to treat your cancer include:

- Three-dimensional conformal radiation therapy (3D-CRT) uses computer software and CT images to aim beams that match the shape of the tumor.
- Intensity-modulated radiation therapy (IMRT) uses small beams of different strengths to match the shape of the tumor.
- Stereotactic body radiation therapy (SBRT) uses high-energy radiation beams to treat cancers in five or fewer treatments.
- Stereotactic radiosurgery (SRS) uses special equipment to position the body and give one precise, large dose of radiation.

Stereotactic body radiation therapy (SBRT) should be done at an experienced high-volume center that has image-guided technology.

Stereotactic body radiation therapy

Stereotactic body radiation therapy (SBRT) is a type of EBRT. It is a treatment option for locally advanced pancreatic cancer and for cancer that has returned after surgery (recurrence).

SBRT may be used to:

- Relieve symptoms such as pain caused by pancreatic cancer metastases
- Treat pancreatic cancer in those who cannot have surgery as a primary treatment due to other health conditions
- Shrink tumors
- Prevent recurrence

With SBRT, you will receive high-dose radiation for 1 to 5 treatments. SBRT is very precise, and thereby reduces the chance of damage to nearby tissues. SBRT should be delivered at an experienced, high-volume center with technology that allows for image-guided radiation therapy or in a clinical trial.

Palliative RT

The goal of palliative RT is to relieve pain and bleeding and/or lessen symptoms. Palliative RT might be used to treat bone metastases that cause pain. It might be given to reduce or lessen symptoms caused by an obstruction or blockage, pain resistant to some medicines, or bleeding. Palliative RT can be an option if you have poor performance status or other serious health issues.

Chemoradiation

Treatment that combines a lower-dose chemotherapy with RT is called chemoradiation. Chemotherapy may improve how well radiation works, and that is why they are sometimes used together.

Types of chemoradiation include:

- Capecitabine with RT (preferred)
- Continuous infusion 5-FU with RT (preferred)
- Gemcitabine with RT

Order of treatments

Most people with pancreatic cancer will receive more than one type of treatment. Next is an overview of the order of treatments and what they do.

- **Neoadjuvant (before)** treatment is given to shrink the tumor before primary treatment (surgery). This might change a borderline resectable tumor into a resectable tumor.
- **Primary treatment** is the main treatment given to rid the body of cancer. Surgery is usually the main treatment for resectable pancreatic cancer.
- **Adjuvant (after) treatment** is given after primary treatment to rid the body of any cancer cells left behind from surgery. It is also used when the risk of cancer returning (recurrence) is felt to be high.
- **First-line treatment** is the first set of treatments given.
- **Second-line treatment** is the next set of treatments given after the first treatment has failed.

Talk to your doctor about your treatment plan and what it means for your stage of pancreatic cancer.

Clinical trials

A clinical trial is a type of medical research study. After being developed and tested in a laboratory, potential new ways of fighting cancer need to be studied in people. If found to be safe and effective in a clinical trial, a drug, device, or treatment approach may be approved by the U.S. Food and Drug Administration (FDA). Everyone with cancer should carefully consider all treatment options available for their cancer type, including standard treatments and clinical trials. Talk to your treatment team about whether a clinical trial might make sense for you.

Phases

Most cancer clinical trials focus on treatment. Treatment trials are done in phases that build on one another.

- **Phase I** trials study the safety and side effects of an investigational drug or treatment approach.
- **Phase II** trials study how well the drug or approach works against a specific type of cancer.
- **Phase III** trials compare the drug or approach to standard treatment. Therefore, some patients will be treated with the new drug or approach and some patients will receive standard treatment. If the results are good, it may be approved by the FDA.
- **Phase IV** trials study the long-term safety and benefit of an FDA-approved treatment.

Finding a clinical trial

In the United States

NCCN Cancer Centers
NCCN.org/cancercenters

The National Cancer Institute (NCI)
cancer.gov/about-cancer/treatment/clinical-trials/search

Worldwide

The U.S. National Library of Medicine (NLM)
clinicaltrials.gov/

Need help finding a clinical trial?
NCI's Cancer Information Service (CIS)
1.800.4.CANCER (1.800.422.6237)
cancer.gov/contact

Who can enroll?

Every clinical trial has rules for joining, called eligibility criteria. The rules may be about age, cancer type and stage, treatment history, or general health. These rules ensure that participants are alike in specific ways and that the treatment is as safe as possible.

Informed consent

Clinical trials are managed by a group of experts called a research team. The research team will review the study with you in detail, including its purpose and the risks and benefits of joining. This information is also described in detail in an informed consent form. Giving informed consent means that you understand the possible benefits and risks and agree to join. Read the form carefully and ask questions before signing it. Take time to discuss with family, friends, or others you trust. Keep in mind that you can leave and seek treatment outside of the clinical trial at any time.

Start the conversation

Don't wait for your doctor to bring up clinical trials. Start the conversation and learn about all of your treatment options. If you find a study that you may be eligible for, ask your treatment team if you meet the requirements. If you already began standard treatment, and then decide to join a clinical trial, you may not be eligible. Try not to be discouraged if you cannot join. New clinical trials are always becoming available.

Frequently asked questions

There are many myths and misconceptions surrounding clinical trials. The possible benefits and risks are not well understood by many with cancer.

What if I get the placebo?

A placebo is an inactive version of a real medicine. Placebos are almost never used alone in cancer clinical trials. All participants receive commonly used (standard) cancer treatment. You may receive a commonly used treatment, the investigational drug, or both.

Do I have to pay to be in a clinical trial?

Rarely. It depends on the study, your health insurance, and the state in which you live. Your treatment team and the research team can help determine if you are responsible for any costs.

Review

- Treatment decisions should involve a multidisciplinary team (MDT) or a team of doctors from different fields of medicine who have knowledge (expertise) and experience with your type of cancer.
- Staging tests are used to measure the size of the primary tumor, to see if and where the cancer has spread, and to look at the pancreas and nearby tissues.
- Pancreatic cancer that can be removed completely with surgery and has not spread outside the pancreas is called resectable.
- When it is unclear if pancreatic cancer can be removed with surgery, it is called borderline resectable.
- Pancreatic cancer that has spread to nearby blood vessels and lymph nodes is called locally advanced. It is unresectable.
- Pancreatic cancer that has spread to distant parts of the body is called metastatic. It is unresectable.
- Performance status (PS) indicates a person's general level of fitness and is used in making treatment decisions.
- Surgery aims to remove the tumor, when possible. The type of surgery you receive depends on size and location of the tumor in the pancreas. It also depends on if there is cancer in any surrounding organs and tissues.
- Chemotherapy kills fast-growing cells throughout the body, including cancer cells and normal cells.

It is important to tell your care team about all of your side effects so they can be managed.

- Targeted therapy focuses on specific or unique features of cancer cells, and sometimes on the presence of genetic mutations in the cancer cells.
- Immunotherapy increases the activity of your immune system.
- Clinical trials study how safe and helpful tests and treatments are for people.

4

Supportive and palliative care

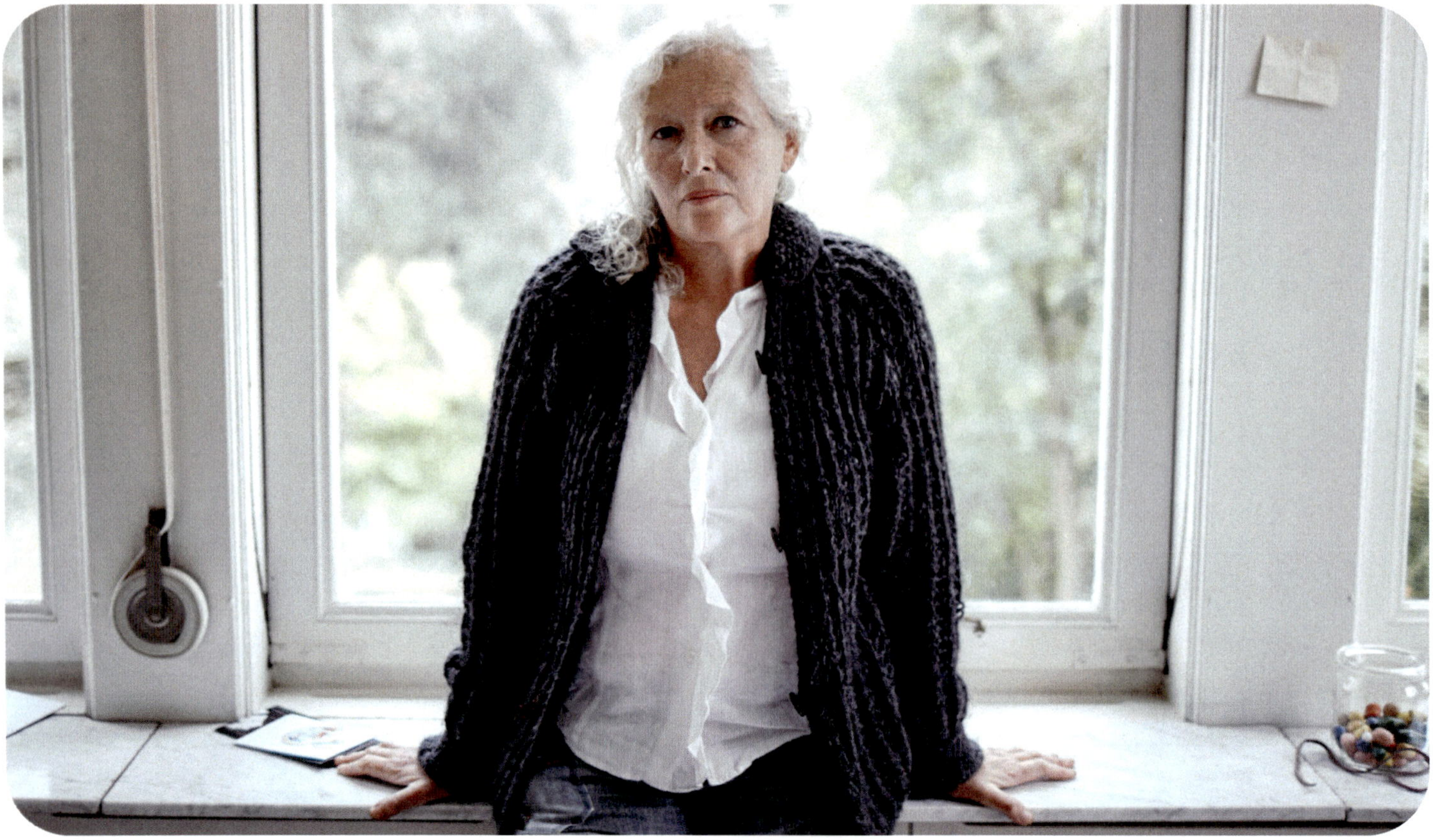

Supportive care is health care that relieves symptoms caused by cancer or its treatment and improves your quality of life.

Overview

Supportive care is health care that relieves symptoms caused by cancer and improves quality of life. It is also referred to as palliative care. Supportive care is recommended for anyone who has symptoms related to pancreatic cancer, or to relieve side effects from treatments for pancreatic cancer.

Supportive care might include pain relief (palliative care), emotional or spiritual support, financial aid, or family counseling. Pancreatic cancer can make it difficult to eat or digest food. These digestive symptoms are also managed through supportive care. Tell your care team how you are feeling and about any side effects.

Best supportive care is used with other treatments to improve quality of life for those with locally advanced and metastatic pancreatic cancer. It is also used when there is cancer recurrence after surgery. Best supportive care, supportive care, and palliative care are often used interchangeably.

Blocked bile duct

A tumor in the pancreas may grow large enough to block your bile duct. A stent is a tiny tube that is placed in the bile duct to unblock it or keep it open.

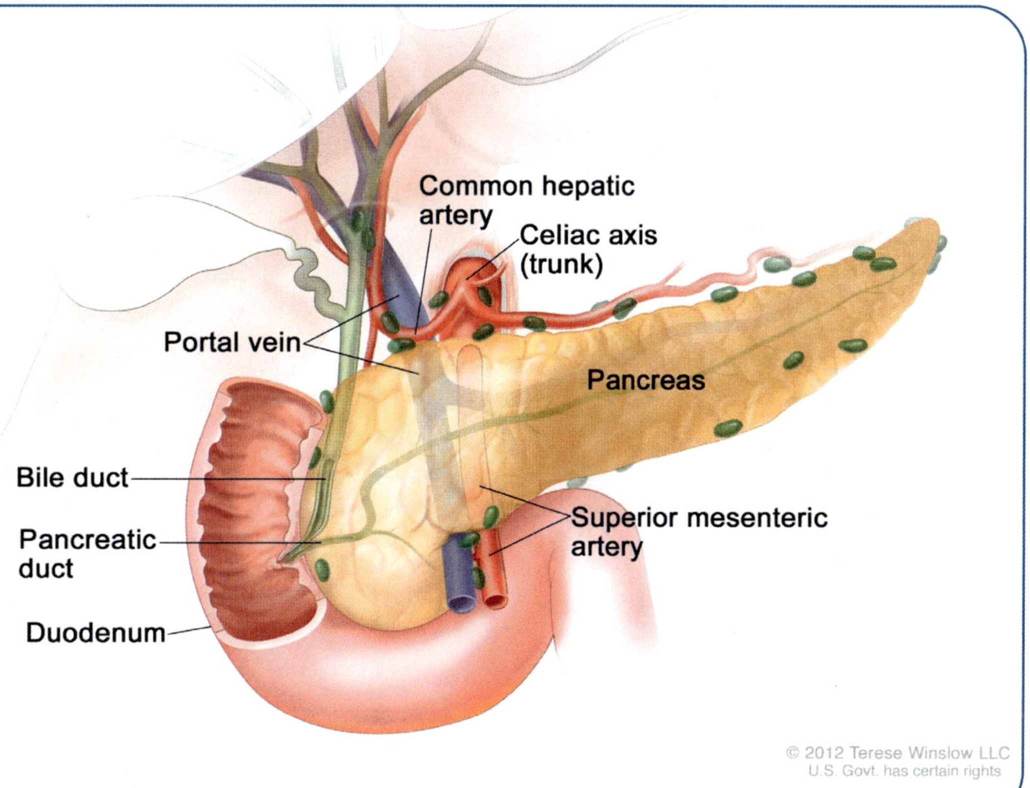

Blocked bile duct

A tumor in the pancreas may grow large enough to block your bile duct. A bile duct is a small tube that drains digestive fluid (bile) from the liver. The common bile duct carries bile from the liver through the pancreas and into the first part of the small intestine (duodenum). A blocked duct causes bile to build up in the liver. As a result, you may have pain, itching, discomfort, dark urine, light-colored stool, and jaundice. This blockage can cause an infection of the bile duct called cholangitis.

A blocked bile duct may be treated by placing a biliary stent (preferred), a biliary drain, or doing a biliary bypass. A biliary stent is a tiny tube that is placed in the bile duct to unblock it or keep it open. Before the stent can be placed with the help of an endoscope, bile may need to be drained through an opening in the side of the body (biliary drain). You may need a new or second stent during or after cancer treatment if the tumor grows. A biliary bypass is a surgery to re-route the flow of bile from the common bile duct into the small intestine. The result is that the bile flow avoids (bypasses) the blocked part of the duct.

Blocked stomach

A tumor in the pancreas may also grow large enough to block food from passing out of your stomach through the first part of the small intestine (duodenum). This blockage can cause pain, vomiting, weight loss, and other problems. Treatments for a blocked stomach include a stent, a PEG (percutaneous endoscopic gastrostomy) tube, or a stomach-duodenum bypass (gastrojejunostomy).

A stent is a tube that expands. It is placed in the small intestine to keep your stomach open so food can pass through. A PEG tube is a tube that is inserted through a cut in the abdomen and placed in the stomach. Food is given through this tube. A gastrojejunostomy is a surgery to re-route the path food takes from the stomach into the small intestine. The new path from the stomach will avoid (bypass) the blocked part of the duodenum. This surgery may also be done as a preventive measure if there is a high risk that your stomach may become blocked.

Blood clots

A blood clot or thrombus is a clump of blood that has changed from a liquid to a gel-like consistency. Blood clots can form in veins. When clots break loose, they can travel to another part of the body and cause serious problems.

Thromboembolic disease is a common complication of pancreatic cancer. Pancreatic cancer cells cause excess platelets to form increasing the chance of blood clots. If you develop a venous thromboembolism (VTE), treatment includes blood thinners (anticoagulants) such as heparin.

Bleeding

The main tumor can cause bleeding in the gastrointestinal (GI) tract. This is rare. An endoscopy, radiation therapy (if not done before), and an angiography with embolization might be used to treat (stop) bleeding.

An angiography is used when a blood vessel is narrowed or if the blood vessel suddenly becomes blocked and does not allow blood to flow. In an angiography, a catheter (thin plastic tube), is inserted into an artery through a small incision in the skin. The catheter is guided to the area with the use of x-rays. A contrast material is injected through the tube and x-ray images produce a picture of the blood vessel called an angiogram.

Embolization is the process of blocking blood flow through a blood vessel. This is performed by placing various materials through the angiography catheter while it is inside the blood vessel. The material can be a coil, small beads, or liquid medicine that causes the blood to clot and block the flow of blood.

Distress

Distress is an unpleasant experience of a mental, physical, social, or spiritual nature. It can affect how you feel, think, and act. Distress might include feelings of sadness, fear, helplessness, worry, anger, and guilt.

Depression, anxiety, and sleeping problems are common in pancreatic cancer. Talk to your doctor and with those whom you feel most comfortable about how you are feeling. There are services and people who can help you. Support and counseling are available. It is recommended that all patients be screened for depression.

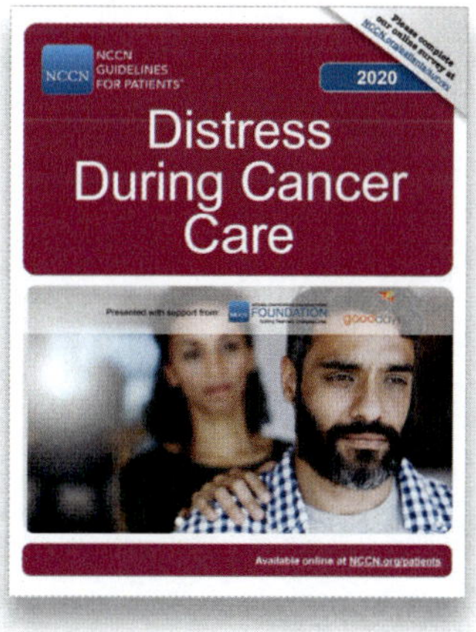

For more information, read *NCCN Guidelines for Patients: Distress During Cancer Care*, available at NCCN.org/patientguidelines.

Diabetes

Diabetes is a condition where the amount of glucose (a type of sugar) in your blood is too high. The amount of glucose in your blood is called your blood sugar level or blood glucose level. If you have diabetes or early-onset diabetes, pancreatic cancer can change how the diabetes is managed. Diabetes can also happen when part or all of your pancreas is removed. Each type of diabetes is different and treated differently.

Exocrine pancreatic insufficiency

Pancreatic cancer or its treatment can cause the pancreas to produce fewer digestive (exocrine) enzymes to break down food. This is called exocrine pancreatic insufficiency (EPI). Symptoms include stomach cramps, gas, loose stools, weight loss, and malnutrition.

Pancreatic enzyme replacement medicine, usually a pill taken by mouth (oral), is given to replace the loss of digestive enzymes. This loss can be caused by surgery, a blocked duct, or from the tumor. You will have trouble digesting food without enough of these enzymes. EPI occurs in most people undergoing surgery. Ask your doctor if you should start enzyme replacement therapy now.

Enzyme replacement therapy can be expensive. Ask your care team if you need help paying for medicine.

Fatigue

Fatigue is extreme tiredness and inability to function due to lack of energy. Fatigue may be caused by pancreatic cancer or it may be a side effect of treatment. There are treatments for fatigue. Let your care team know how you are feeling and if fatigue is getting in the way of doing the things you enjoy. Eating a balanced diet, exercise, yoga, and massage therapy can help. You might be referred to a nutritionist or dietitian to help with fatigue.

Trouble eating and weight loss

Sometimes side effects from surgery, pancreatic cancer, or its treatment might cause you to feel not hungry (low appetite) or sick to your stomach (nauseated). You might have abdominal cramps or trouble digesting food. Healthy eating is important during treatment. It includes eating a balanced diet, eating the right amount of food, and drinking enough fluids. A registered dietitian who is an expert in nutrition and food can help. Speak to your care team if you have trouble eating or maintaining weight.

Nausea and vomiting

Nausea and vomiting are a common side effect of treatment. You will be given medicine to prevent and treat nausea and vomiting.

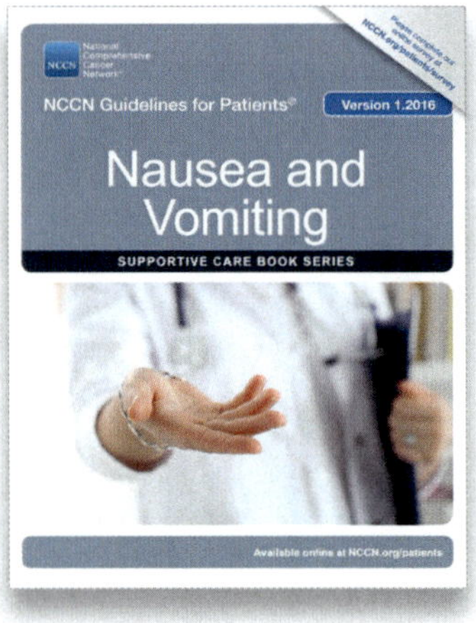

For more information, read the *NCCN Guidelines for Patients: Nausea and Vomiting,* available at NCCN.org/patientguidelines.

Pain

Tell your care team about any pain or discomfort. You might meet with a palliative care specialist or with a pain specialist to manage pain.

Pain is common in those with localized and metastatic pancreatic cancer. Severe abdominal pain can occur when the tumor grows into nearby nerves or presses against other organs. This pain is treated with around-the-clock medicine such as morphine or other opioids (narcotics). Sometimes, non-narcotic medicines are used to treat pain.

When severe abdominal pain no longer responds to pain medicine or the medicine is causing side effects, there are 2 options:

- EUS-guided or percutaneous (injection through the skin) nerve block (celiac plexus neurolysis)
- Palliative radiation with or without systemic therapy

An EUS-guided celiac plexus neurolysis is a nerve block. It uses an endoscope to place a needle into the pancreatic tumor. Other times, an anesthesia pain doctor may perform the nerve block through the skin (percutaneous) in your back directly into the pancreatic tumor. These injections are given to the nerves that transmit pain from the pancreas to the brain. This blocks the pain.

Some may benefit from palliative radiation therapy, with or without systemic therapy, to help relieve the pain. During this treatment, a radiation beam is focused on the tumor.

Keep a pain diary

A pain diary is a written record that helps you keep track of when you have pain, how bad it is, what causes it, and what makes it better or worse. Use a pain diary to discuss your pain with your care team. You might be referred to a specialist for pain management.

Include in your pain diary:

- The time and dose of all medicines
- When pain starts and ends or lessens
- Where you feel pain
- Describe your pain. Is it throbbing, sharp, tingling, shooting, or burning? Is it constant, or does it come and go?
- Does the pain change at different times of day? When?
- Does the pain get worse before or after meals? Does certain food or drink make it better?
- Does the pain get better or worse with activity? What kind of activity?
- Does the pain keep you from falling asleep at night? Does pain wake you up in the night?
- Rate your pain from 0 (no pain) to 10 (worst pain you have ever felt)
- Does pain get in the way of doing the things you enjoy?

Ask questions and seek information about supportive and palliative care options for your pain. Keeping a pain diary can help.

Other side effects

All cancer treatments can cause unwanted health issues called side effects. Side effects depend on many factors. These factors include the drug type and dose, length of treatment, and the person. Some side effects may be harmful to your health. Others may just be unpleasant. Some common side effects are described next.

Diarrhea

Diarrhea is frequent and watery bowel movements. Your care team will tell you how to manage diarrhea and may recommend medicines to stop the diarrhea. It is important to drink lots of fluids.

Infection

You will be monitored for infection. In neutropenia, a low number of white blood cells can lead to frequent or severe infections. When someone with neutropenia also develops a fever, it is called febrile neutropenia (FN). With FN, your risk of infection may be higher than normal. This is because a low number of white blood cells leads to a reduced ability to fight infections. FN is a side effect of some types of chemotherapy.

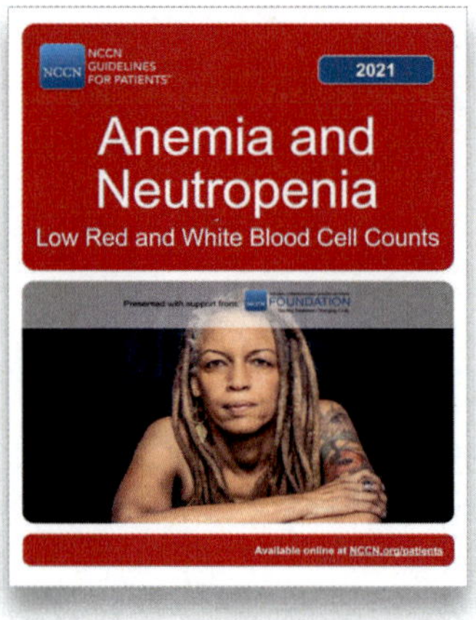

For more information, read the *NCCN Guidelines for Patients: Anemia and Neutropenia,* available at NCCN.org/patientguidelines.

Hand-foot syndrome

Hand-foot syndrome is a common side effect of chemotherapy. It occurs when small amounts of chemotherapy leak out of very small blood vessels called capillaries in the palms of the hands and soles of the feet. It causes redness, swelling, and pain. Sometimes blisters appear. You will want to protect your hands and feet by applying moisturizer or lotion, using gloves when washing dishes, and spreading yard work over several days.

Neuropathy

Neuropathy is a nerve problem that causes pain, numbness, tingling, swelling, or muscle weakness in different parts of the body. It usually begins in the hands or feet and gets worse over time. Neuropathy may be caused by cancer or cancer treatment.

Neurotoxicity

Some treatments can damage the nervous system (neurotoxicity) causing problems with concentration and memory. Seizures and confusion can occur.

Advance care planning

Advance care planning makes decisions now about your care and how you would want to be treated if you become unable to speak for yourself. Advance care planning is for everyone, not just for those who are very sick. It is a way to ensure your wishes are understood and respected.

Advance care planning starts with an honest discussion with your doctor. Ask your doctor about the course your cancer will take called a cancer prognosis. Find out what you might expect if your cancer spreads. Discuss the medicines or therapies that will give you the best quality of life. Include family and friends in your advance care planning. Make your wishes clear. It is important that everyone understands what you want.

You don't have to know the exact details of your prognosis. Just having a general idea will help with planning. With this information, you can decide if there is a point you might want to stop cancer treatment. You can also decide what treatments you would want for symptom relief, such as radiation therapy, surgery, or medicine.

You can change your advance care plan at any time. It might be helpful to have this talk with your doctor and/or friends and family more than once during your treatment. Make your wishes clear; this will ensure everyone knows what you want.

Need help paying for medicine or treatment?

Ask your care team what options are available.

Review

- Supportive care is health care that relieves symptoms caused by cancer or its treatment and improves quality of life. Supportive care is always given.
- All cancer treatments can cause unwanted health issues called side effects. It is important for you to tell your care team about all of your side effects.
- A stent is a tiny tube that may be used to unblock a bile duct or the stomach. Surgery is also a treatment used to unblock or bypass a bile duct or the stomach.
- Pancreatic cancer cells may increase the chance of blood clots, which will need to be treated with blood thinners.
- Pancreatic enzyme replacement therapy, usually a pill taken by mouth (oral), is given to replace the loss of digestive enzymes. The loss of digestive enzymes can cause stomach cramping, gas, loose stools, and weight loss.
- Healthy eating is important during treatment. It includes eating a balanced diet, eating the right amount of food, and drinking enough fluids.
- Pain may be treated with medication, a nerve block, or radiation with or without systemic therapy. A pain diary might help you manage pain.
- A registered dietitian who is an expert in nutrition and food can help if it is hard for you to eat or digest food.
- Advance care planning starts with an honest talk between you and your doctor.

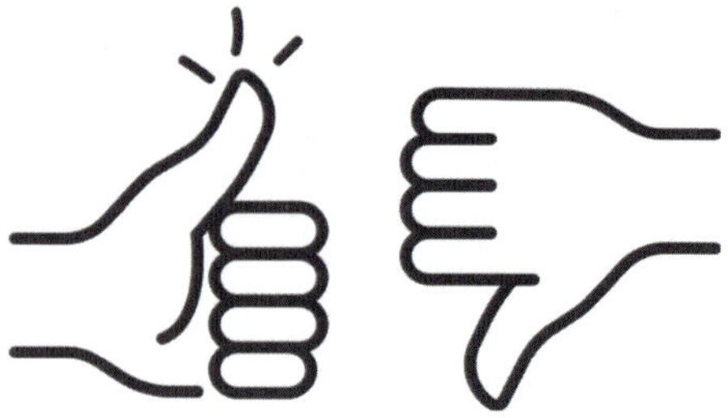

Let us know what you think!

Please take a moment to complete an online survey about the NCCN Guidelines for Patients.

NCCN.org/patients/response

5 Resectable

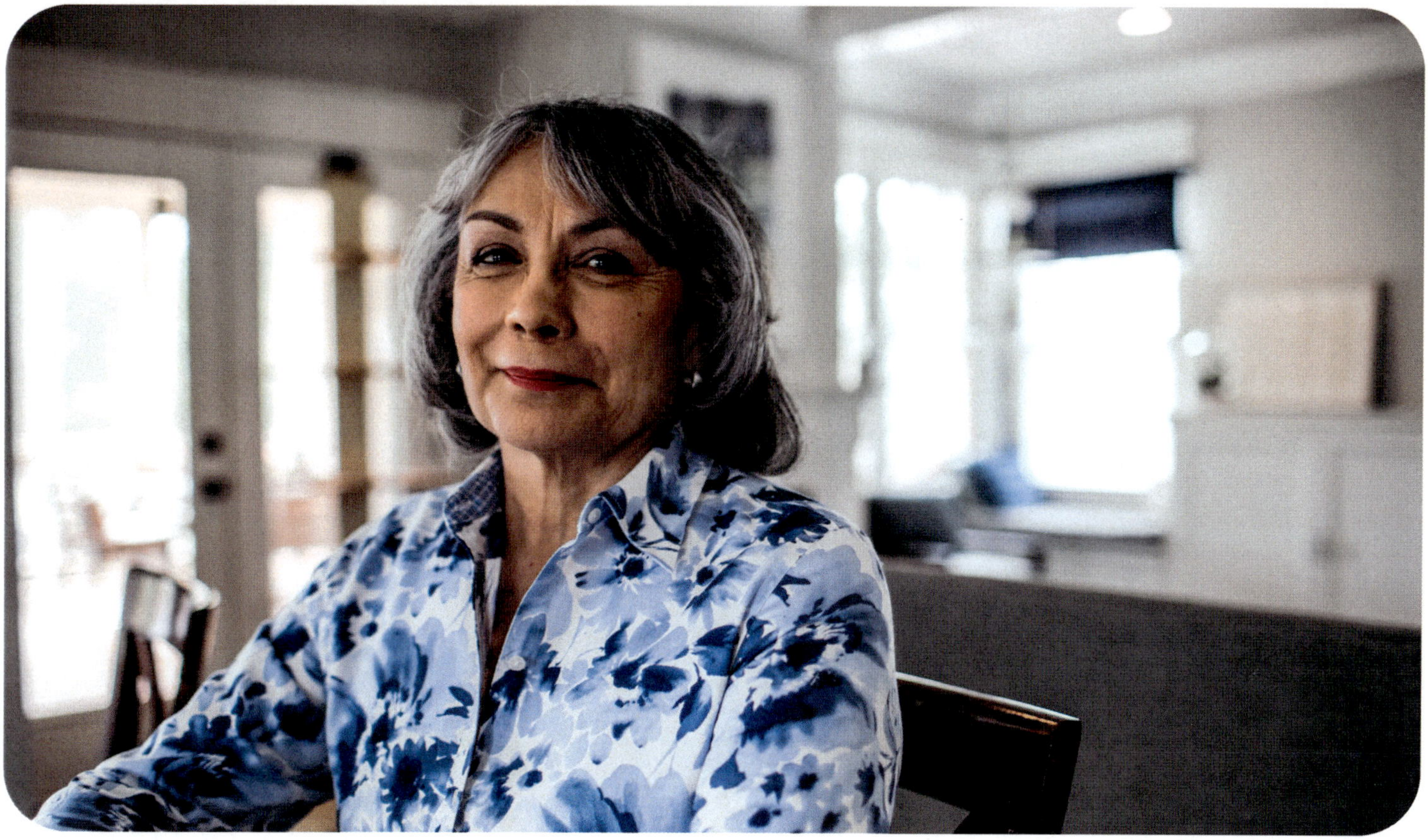

Resectable cancer is found only in the pancreas and can be removed completely with surgery. Together, you and your doctor will choose a treatment plan that is best for you.

Surgery is the primary treatment for resectable pancreatic cancer. Primary treatment refers to the first or main treatment used to treat cancer. Sometimes, treatment is given before surgery to help shrink the tumor. This is called neoadjuvant therapy.

Before surgery

Neoadjuvant therapy might be given in some cases or if you have high-risk features. High-risk features include imaging findings, very highly elevated CA 19-9, large primary tumors, large regional lymph nodes, excessive weight loss, and extreme pain. If you and your doctor are considering neoadjuvant therapy, treatment at a clinic or hospital that specializes in pancreatic cancer is preferred, when possible. Systemic therapy and, sometimes, chemoradiation are possible neoadjuvant therapies for resectable pancreatic cancer. See Guide 5.

A laparoscopy might be done to stage your cancer before starting treatment.

There are 2 treatment options for resectable cancer:

- Surgery followed by adjvant therapy
- Neoadjuvant therapy before surgery

Neoadjuvant therapy

Before starting neoadjuvant therapy, you might have an EUS-guided biopsy and/or stent placement.

After neoadjuvant therapy, you will have a:

- Repeat pancreatic protocol CT or MRI
- Repeat chest/pelvic CT
- CA 19-9 test

Guide 5 Neoadjuvant therapy options: Resectable disease
FOLFIRINOX or modified FOLFIRINOX (for those with PS 0 or 1)
Gemcitabine with albumin-bound paclitaxel
Only for known *BRCA1, BRCA2,* or *PALB2* mutations: • FOLFIRINOX or modified FOLFIRINOX (for those with PS 0 or 1) • Gemcitabine with cisplatin

* All options might be followed with chemoradiation

A high CA 19-9 does not necessarily mean there is cancer. CA 19-9 may be elevated from biliary infection (cholangitis), inflammation, or an obstruction.

Surgery

Surgery to remove the tumor can be open or minimally invasive. A team of doctors will need to agree that surgery is the best choice in your case. When deciding if surgery is possible, your doctor should work with a team of experts at a hospital that does more than 15 to 20 pancreatic cancer surgeries each year. This is considered a high-volume center.

Pancreatic surgery is complex. You want an experienced surgeon who can make difficult decisions during surgery. If the tumor has grown into veins and arteries in such a way that makes it unsafe to remove, your resectable pancreatic cancer is now called unresectable.

Cancer found unresectable

If during surgery, it is determined that your tumor cannot be removed safely, then a biopsy will be done to confirm pancreatic cancer. Other procedures might be done at this time based on if there is or isn't jaundice. Treatment options will follow Chapter 7: Locally advanced or Chapter 8: Metastatic disease.

If there isn't jaundice, you might have:

- Gastrojejunostomy
- Celiac plexus neurolysis, if you have pain

If there is jaundice, you might have:

- Biliary bypass or stent
- Gastrojejunostomy
- Celiac plexus neurolysis if you have pain

Biliary bypass or stent

If you have or are at risk of developing jaundice, you might have a biliary bypass to re-route the flow of bile around the blocked part of the bile duct. A stent might be placed if you have a blocked bile duct.

Gastrojejunostomy

In a duodenal bypass (gastrojejunostomy), a path is created between the stomach and the middle section of the small intestine. It may be done if cancer is blocking the stomach or the first part of the small intestine (duodenum). The new path from the stomach will avoid (bypass) the blocked part of the duodenum. This surgery may be used as a preventive measure if there is a high risk that your stomach may become blocked.

Celiac plexus neurolysis

If you have severe pain, the surgeon may inject alcohol (ethanol) and an anesthetic such as bupivacaine into the nerves around the pancreatic cancer (celiac plexus). These nerves are destroyed in order to relieve the pain. This nerve block is referred to as celiac plexus neurolysis.

After surgery

Adjuvant therapy is treatment given after surgery to rid the body of cancer cells and to help prevent recurrence. If surgery is successful and all of the tumor can be removed, you will have adjuvant therapy.

Before beginning adjuvant therapy, you will have a CA 19-9 blood test and CT scan with contrast of the chest, pelvis, and abdomen. These tests are done to check for signs of recurrence and metastasis, and will serve as a baseline for future tests. You will have germline testing if it hasn't been done before.

If tests find metastases

If tests show metastases, see Chapter 8: Metastatic disease.

If tests find no metastases

If the tests do not show any signs of metastases or recurrence, then you will receive adjuvant therapy. Adjuvant therapy should only be started after you've fully recovered from surgery, but within 12 weeks after surgery.

The options for adjuvant treatment are based on if you had neoadjuvant therapy before surgery. If you did not have neoadjuvant therapy, then a clinical trial is preferred. Adjuvant therapy options are based on the tumor's response to neoadjuvant therapy and other factors. For treatment options, see Guide 6 and Guide 7.

Monitoring

After treatment you will be monitored for recurrence. If cancer returns, it is called recurrence.

You will have the following tests as needed every 3 to 6 months for 2 years, then every 6 to 12 months:

- Medical history and physical exam to assess symptoms
- CA 19-9 level
- Chest CT and CT or MRI of abdomen and pelvis with contrast

Guide 6
Adjuvant therapy options: Resectable disease

No, I did not have neoadjuvant therapy before surgery	• Clinical trial (preferred) • Chemotherapy alone • Chemotherapy, then chemoradiation. This might be followed by more lines of chemotherapy.
Yes, I had neoadjuvant therapy before surgery	• Chemotherapy and/or • Chemoradiation in a positive margin R1 resection

Recurrence after surgery

For recurrence, you might have the following:

- Biopsy to confirm recurrence
- Genetic (germline) testing, if not done before
- Biomarker (tumor) testing, if not done before

MSI and/or MMR testing can be done as part of germline or gene profile testing.

Local recurrence

If cancer returns to the pancreas, you should have a surgical consult and a multidisciplinary team review to determine if surgery is an option.

If cancer returns to the operative bed, the options are:

- Clinical trial (preferred)
- Systemic therapy (see Guide 8)
- Systemic therapy followed by chemoradiation or SBRT (if not done before)
- SBRT
- Palliative and best supportive care

Chemoradiation or SBRT might be done in some people who aren't candidates for systemic therapy. SBRT is a type of radiation therapy. Chemotherapies used in chemoradiation include capecitabine, continuous infusion 5-FU, or gemcitabine.

Guide 7
Adjuvant systemic therapy options

Preferred options	• Modified FOLFIRINOX (for those with PS 0 or 1) • Gemcitabine with capecitabine
Other recommended	• Gemcitabine • 5-FU with leucovorin • Continuous infusion 5-FU • Capecitabine • Gemcitabine followed by chemoradiation • 5-FU with leucovorin followed by chemoradiation • Continuous infusion 5-FU followed by chemoradiation • Gemcitabine followed by chemoradiation and then gemcitabine • 5-FU with leucovorin followed by chemoradiation and then 5-FU with leucovorin • Continuous infusion 5-FU followed by chemoradiation and then continuous infusion 5-FU

Metastatic recurrence

Pancreatic cancer can spread to the liver, lungs, abdominal cavity, and other areas of the body. Treatment options are based on the length of time since completing primary therapy. A clinical trial is preferred. For all options, see Guide 8.

A clinical trial is preferred when cancer returns after surgery.

Guide 8
Treatment options: Local and metastatic recurrence

6 months or more have passed since finishing primary therapy	• Clinical trial (preferred) • Repeat systemic therapy used before • Systemic therapy not used before • Palliative and best supportive care
Less than 6 months have passed since finishing primary therapy	• Clinical trial (preferred) • Switch to gemcitabine-based systemic chemotherapy (if fluoropyrimidine-based therapy used before) • Switch to fluoropyrimidine-based systemic chemotherapy (if gemcitabine-based therapy used before) • Palliative and best supportive care

Review

- Pancreatic cancer that can be removed completely with surgery and has not spread outside the pancreas is called resectable.
- In resectable pancreatic cancer, surgery is used as the primary treatment to remove the tumor. You might have neoadjuvant therapy before surgery to shrink the tumor and reduce the amount of cancer cells.
- If the tumor was removed (resected) during surgery, then you will have adjuvant therapy to rid the body of cancer cells and to help prevent recurrence. Options are based on if you had neoadjuvant therapy before surgery.
- If your surgeon was unable to remove your tumor, it is now called unresectable. Biopsies and other tests will be done to see if the cancer is locally advanced or metastatic.
- Adjuvant therapy should only be started after you've fully recovered from surgery, but within 12 weeks after surgery.
- After finishing adjuvant therapy, you will go through follow-up testing and be monitored for recurrence.
- If cancer returns after surgery, treatment will be based on if it is a local or metastatic recurrence.
- If cancer has returned or metastasized, treatment is based on how long it has been since primary therapy ended.

Systemic therapy is used in all stages of pancreatic cancer. Goals of systemic therapy should be discussed.

6

Borderline resectable

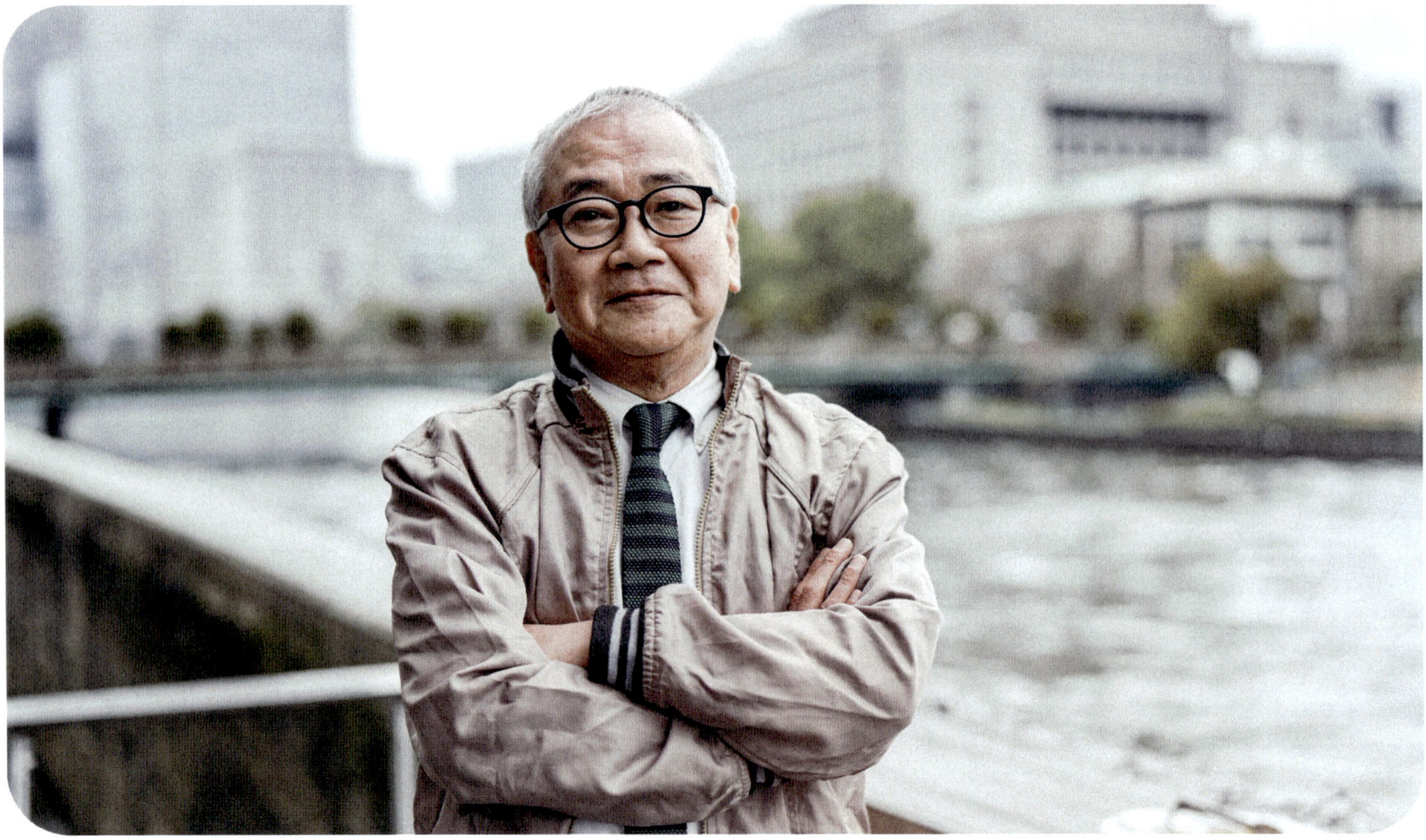

Borderline resectable cancer is found in the pancreas and might involve nearby veins and arteries. Together, you and your doctor will choose a treatment plan that is best for you.

Overview

In borderline resectable cancer, the cancer is found only in the pancreas but might involve nearby blood vessels or structures. When the tumor is wrapped around part of the hepatic artery, superior mesenteric artery, or superior mesenteric vein, and there is risk for a positive margin, then surgery might not be the best option.

For borderline resectable cancer, you should receive treatment before surgery called neoadjuvant therapy. The goal of neoadjuvant therapy is to try to shrink the tumor in order to make it easier to remove during surgery.

Arteries and veins in and near the pancreas

When the tumor is wrapped around part of the hepatic artery, superior mesenteric artery, or superior mesenteric vein, and there is risk for a positive margin, then surgery might not be the best option.

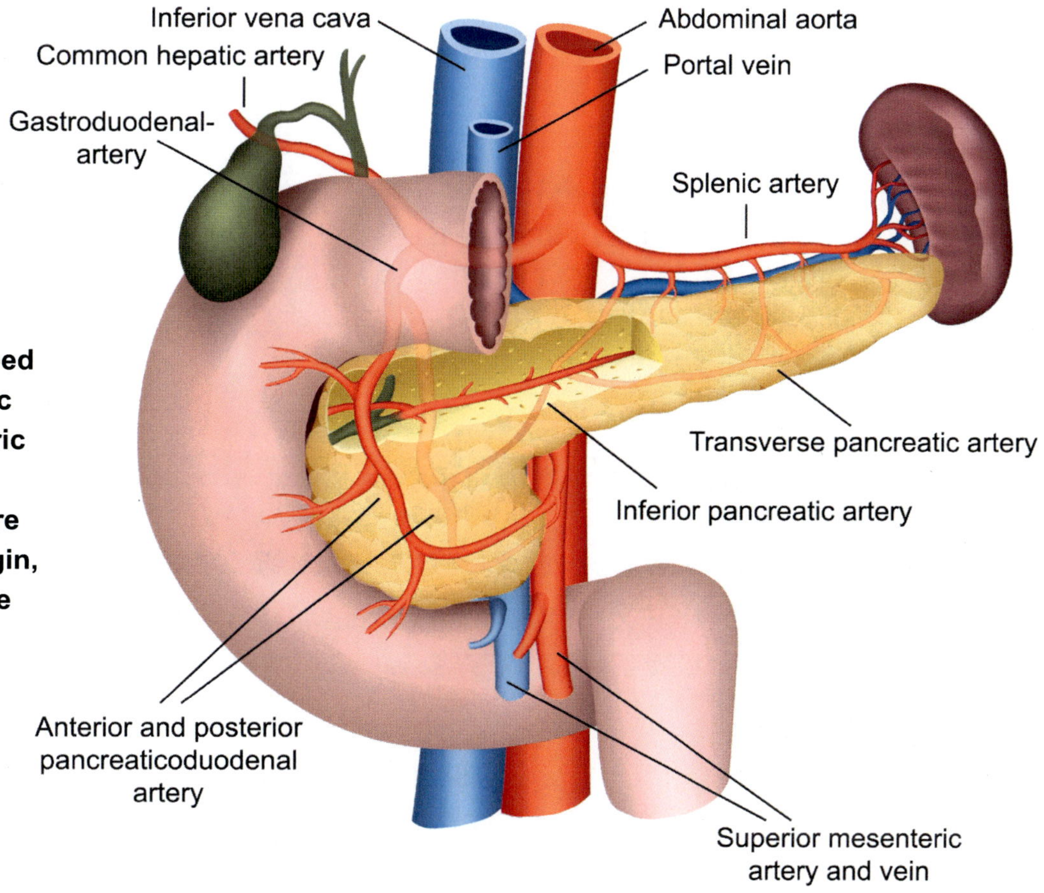

Tests

Before treatment, you will have a biopsy. An EUS-guided fine-needle aspiration (FNA) is preferred. A baseline CA 19-9 will be done and you might have a staging laparoscopy.

Cancer cannot be confirmed

If cancer cannot be confirmed, you will have a repeat biopsy. If pancreatic cancer still cannot be confirmed, then you will be referred to a high-volume center for evaluation.

Cancer confirmed

If cancer is confirmed, you might have an ERCP with stent placement before starting neoadjuvant therapy. Neoadjuvant therapy is given before surgery.

Before surgery

Treatment before surgery is called neoadjuvant therapy. The goal of neoadjuvant therapy is to try to shrink the tumor in order to make it easier to remove during surgery. It might not be possible to shrink the tumor or the amount of cancer.

If you and your doctor are considering neoadjuvant therapy, treatment at a hospital that specializes in pancreatic cancer is preferred, when possible. Systemic therapy with or without chemoradiation are possible neoadjuvant therapies for borderline resectable pancreatic cancer. See Guide 9.

After neoadjuvant therapy, you will have a:

- Pancreatic protocol CT or MRI of abdomen
- Chest/pelvic CT
- CA 19-9 test

If surgery is possible, then you might have a staging laparoscopy before surgery.

If cancer has progressed or spread, then you will not have surgery. Treatment options will follow *Chapter 7: Locally advanced or Chapter 8: Metastatic disease*.

Guide 9 Neoadjuvant therapy options: Borderline resectable disease
FOLFIRINOX or modified FOLFIRINOX (for those with PS 0 or 1)
Gemcitabine with albumin-bound paclitaxel
Only for known *BRCA1, BRCA2,* or *PALB2* mutations: • FOLFIRINOX or modified FOLFIRINOX (for those with PS 0 or 1) • Gemcitabine with cisplatin

* All options might be followed with chemoradiation

Surgery

Pancreatic surgery is complex. You want an experienced surgeon who can make difficult decisions during surgery. When deciding if surgery is possible, your doctor should work with a team of experts at a hospital that does more than 15 to 20 pancreatic cancer surgeries each year. This is considered a high-volume center.

Cancer found unresectable

If during surgery it is determined that your tumor cannot be removed safely, then a biopsy of the tumor will be done if not done before. Other procedures might be done at this time based on if there is or isn't jaundice. Treatment options will follow *Chapter 7: Locally advanced or Chapter 8: Metastatic disease.*

If there isn't jaundice, you may have:

- Gastrojejunostomy
- Celiac plexus neurolysis, if you have pain

If there is jaundice, you may have:

- Biliary bypass or stent
- Gastrojejunostomy
- Celiac plexus neurolysis, if you have pain

Biliary bypass or stent

If you have or are at risk of developing jaundice, you might have a biliary bypass to re-route the flow of bile around the blocked part of the bile duct. A stent might be placed if you have a blocked bile duct.

Gastrojejunostomy

In a duodenal bypass (gastrojejunostomy), a path is created between the stomach and the middle section of the small intestine. It may be done if cancer is blocking the stomach or the first part of the small intestine (duodenum). The new path from the stomach will avoid (bypass) the blocked part of the duodenum. This surgery may be used as a preventive measure if there is a high risk that your stomach may become blocked.

Celiac plexus neurolysis

If you have severe pain, the surgeon may inject alcohol (ethanol) and an anesthetic such as bupivacaine into the nerves around the pancreatic cancer (celiac plexus). These nerves are destroyed in order to relieve the pain. This nerve block is referred to as celiac plexus neurolysis.

After surgery

Adjuvant therapy is treatment given after surgery to rid the body of cancer cells and to help prevent recurrence. If all of the tumor was removed during surgery and you did not complete all chemotherapy before surgery, then you may have adjuvant therapy.

Options include:

- Clinical trial (preferred)
- Chemotherapy alone
- Chemotherapy, then chemoradiation. This might be followed by more lines of chemotherapy.

Before beginning adjuvant therapy, you will have a CA 19-9 blood test and CT scan with contrast of the chest, pelvis, and abdomen. These tests are done to check for signs of recurrence and metastasis, and will serve as a baseline for future tests. You will have germline testing if it hasn't been done before.

For chemotherapy options, see Guide 10.

Guide 10
Adjuvant chemotherapy options

Preferred options	• Modified FOLFIRINOX (for those with PS 0 or 1) • Gemcitabine with capecitabine
Other recommended	• Gemcitabine • 5-FU with leucovorin • Continuous infusion 5-FU • Capecitabine • Gemcitabine followed by chemoradiation • 5-FU with leucovorin followed by chemoradiation • Continuous infusion 5-FU followed by chemoradiation • Gemcitabine followed by chemoradiation and then gemcitabine • 5-FU with leucovorin followed by chemoradiation and then 5-FU with leucovorin • Continuous infusion 5-FU followed by chemoradiation and then continuous infusion 5-FU

Recurrence after surgery

For cancer that returns after surgery, you might have a biopsy to confirm recurrence and, if not done before, genetic (germline) and biomarker (tumor) testing.

Local recurrence

In local recurrence, cancer has returned to the pancreas or the surgical bed. When part or all of the pancreas has been removed, the area that remains is called the surgical or operative bed. Cancer may return to this area. This is treated differently than cancer that has returned to the pancreas or cancer that has spread (metastasized) to distant sites in the body.

If cancer returns to the pancreas, you should have a surgical consult with a multidisciplinary review to determine if surgery is an option.

For cancer that has returned to the operative bed, the options are:

- Clinical trial (preferred)
- Systemic therapy
- Systemic therapy followed by chemoradiation or SBRT (if not done before)
- SBRT
- Palliative and best supportive care

Chemoradiation or SBRT might be done in some people who aren't candidates for systemic therapy. SBRT is a type of radiation therapy. Chemotherapies used in chemoradiation include capecitabine, continuous infusion 5-FU, or gemcitabine.

Guide 11
Treatment options: Recurrence after surgery

6 months or more have passed since finishing primary therapy	• Clinical trial (preferred) • Repeat systemic therapy used before • Systemic therapy not used before • Palliative and best supportive care
Less than 6 months have passed since finishing primary therapy	• Clinical trial (preferred) • Switch to gemcitabine-based systemic chemotherapy (if fluoropyrimidine-based therapy used before) • Switch to fluoropyrimidine-based systemic chemotherapy (if gemcitabine-based therapy used before) • Palliative and best supportive care

Metastatic recurrence

Pancreatic cancer can spread to the liver, lungs, abdominal cavity, and other areas of the body. Treatment options are based on the length of time since completing primary therapy. A clinical trial is preferred. See Guide 11.

For possible second-line therapy options, see Guide 12.

Guide 12
Second-line systemic therapy options

If you had gemcitabine-based therapy before	• 5-FU with leucovorin and liposomal irinotecan • 5-FU with leucovorin and irinotecan (FOLFIRI) • FOLFIRINOX or modified FOLFIRINOX • Oxaliplatin with 5-FU and leucovorin (OFF) • FOLFOX • Capecitabine with oxaliplatin • Capecitabine • Continuous infusion 5-FU
If you had fluoropyrimidine-based therapy before	• Gemcitabine • Gemcitabine with albumin-bound paclitaxel • Gemcitabine with cisplatin (only for known *BRCA1, BRCA2,* or *PALB2* mutations) • Gemcitabine with erlotinib • 5-FU with leucovorin and liposomal irinotecan (if no prior irinotecan)
Used in some cases	• Pembrolizumab (only for MSI-H or dMMR tumors) • Larotrectinib (if *NTRK* gene fusion-positive) • Entrectinib (if *NTRK* gene fusion-positive)

Review

- In borderline resectable cancer, the cancer is found only in the pancreas but might involve nearby blood vessels or structures. Surgery may not be possible.
- Treatment before surgery is called neoadjuvant therapy. The goal of neoadjuvant therapy is to try to shrink the tumor in order make it easier to remove during surgery. Everyone should receive neoadjuvant therapy.
- Treatment after surgery is called adjuvant therapy. The goal of adjuvant therapy is to kill any remaining cancerous cells and to help prevent cancer returning (recurrence).
- Sometimes, during surgery it is discovered that your tumor cannot be removed safely (unresectable). At this time, you might have a biliary bypass, a stent, a duodenal bypass, and/or a nerve block.
- In a duodenal bypass (gastrojejunostomy), a path is created between the stomach and the middle section of the small intestine.
- If you have or are at risk of developing jaundice, you might have a biliary bypass to re-route the flow of bile around the blocked part of the bile duct. A stent might be placed if you have a blocked bile duct.
- If cancer returns after surgery, treatment will be based on if it is a local or metastatic recurrence.

A clinical trial is preferred when cancer returns after surgery.

7 Locally advanced

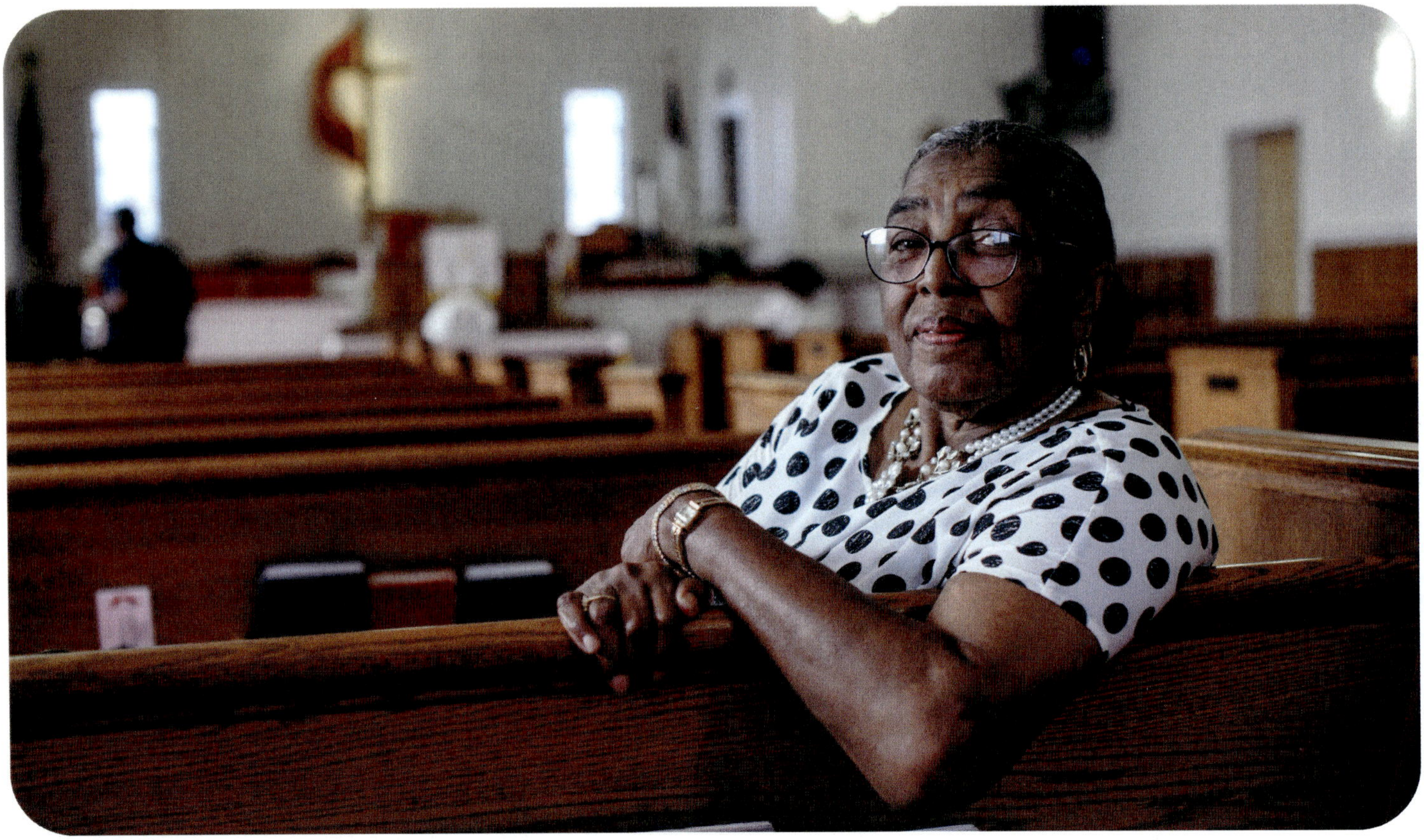

Locally advanced cancer that has spread outside the pancreas to nearby blood vessels, lymph nodes, or other tissues. Together, you and your doctor will choose a treatment plan that is best for you.

Tests

If not done before, you will have a biopsy before starting treatment. This is to confirm pancreatic cancer.

Cancer cannot be confirmed

If cancer cannot be confirmed, you will have a repeat biopsy. For jaundice, an ERCP with stent placement might be done. If pancreatic cancer still cannot be confirmed with a biopsy, then you will be referred to a high-volume center for evaluation.

Cancer confirmed

If cancer is confirmed, then you might have:

- If not done before, genetic (germline) and biomarker (tumor) testing

For jaundice, an ERCP with stent placement might be done.

First-line therapy

First-line treatment is the first treatment or set of treatments given to control the cancer. It is based on performance status (PS). The goal of treatment is to prevent or delay disease progression and to control the spread of disease.

Poor PS

Poor PS is PS 2, PS 3, or PS 4. Palliative and best supportive care are always given for those with poor PS. In addition, you might be given chemotherapy or palliative radiation therapy (RT).

Preferred chemotherapy options include:

- Gemcitabine
- Capecitabine
- Continuous infusion 5-FU

Targeted therapies used in some cases:

- Pembrolizumab (only for MSI-H or dMMR tumors)
- If *NTRK* gene fusion-positive, then larotrectinib or entrectinib

Good PS

Good PS is usually PS 0 or PS 1 with good biliary drainage and adequate nutritional intake.

First-line therapy options for good PS include:

- Clinical trial (preferred)
- Systemic therapy, see Guide 13
- Chemotherapy followed by chemoradiation or stereotactic body radiation therapy (SBRT)
- Chemoradiation or SBRT

Radiation therapy

The goal of RT in locally advanced pancreatic cancer is to prevent or delay disease progression and to control the spread of disease. It is also used for pain or discomfort caused by blockages.

Chemoradiation

Treatment that combines chemotherapy with radiation therapy (RT) is called chemoradiation.

Guide 13
First-line systemic therapy options: Locally advanced disease with good PS

Preferred options	• FOLFIRINOX or modified FOLFIRINOX (for those with PS 0 or 1) • Gemcitabine with albumin-bound paclitaxel
	Only for known *BRCA1, BRCA2,* or *PALB2* mutations: • FOLFIRINOX or modified FOLFIRINOX • Gemcitabine with cisplatin
Other recommended	• Gemcitabine with erlotinib • Gemcitabine with capecitabine • Gemcitabine • Capecitabine • Continuous infusion 5-FU • Fixed-dose-rate gemcitabine, docetaxel, capecitabine (GTX regimen) • Fluoropyrimidine with oxaliplatin
Used in some cases	• Chemotherapy with any of the preferred or other recommended regimens followed by chemoradiation or SBRT • Chemoradiation or SBRT

After first-line therapy

After first-line therapy, your performance status (PS) will be assessed. Next steps will be based on your PS and if disease has progressed. Good PS is usually PS 0 or PS 1 with good biliary drainage and adequate nutritional intake. Your care team will look for signs of disease progression and monitor your PS throughout treatment.

Guide 14
Second-line systemic therapy options: Locally advanced disease with good PS

If you had gemcitabine-based therapy before	• 5-FU with leucovorin and liposomal irinotecan • 5-FU with leucovorin and irinotecan (FOLFIRI) • FOLFIRINOX or modified FOLFIRINOX • Oxaliplatin with 5-FU and leucovorin (OFF) • FOLFOX • Capecitabine with oxaliplatin • Capecitabine • Continuous infusion 5-FU
If you had fluoropyrimidine-based therapy before	• Gemcitabine • Gemcitabine with albumin-bound paclitaxel • Gemcitabine with cisplatin (only for known *BRCA1, BRCA2,* or *PALB2* mutations) • Gemcitabine with erlotinib • 5-FU with leucovorin and liposomal irinotecan (if no prior irinotecan)
Used in some cases	• Pembrolizumab (only for MSI-H or dMMR tumors) • Larotrectinib (if *NTRK* gene fusion-positive) • Entrectinib (if *NTRK* gene fusion-positive)

Good PS with disease progression

If disease has progressed and you have good PS, then the treatment options are:

- Clinical trial (preferred)
- Systemic therapy, see Guide 14
- Chemoradiation
- SBRT, if not previously given and if primary site is the only site of progression

If disease continues to progress with good PS, then a clinical trial would be next. If PS starts declining, then you will begin palliative and supportive care.

Good PS without disease progression

If disease hasn't progressed and you have good PS, then the treatment options are:

- Surgery (resection), if possible. Might be followed with adjuvant therapy
- Observation followed by monitoring for disease progression
- Continue systemic therapy
- Clinical trial

Poor PS with disease progression

If disease has progressed, then the treatment options are:

- Palliative and best supportive care
- Chemotherapy or possibly targeted therapy
- Palliative RT

Preferred chemotherapy options include gemcitabine, capecitabine, or continuous infusion 5-FU.

Targeted therapies used in some cases:

- Pembrolizumab (only for MSI-H or dMMR tumors)
- If *NTRK* gene fusion-positive, then larotrectinib or entrectinib

Review

- In locally advanced pancreatic cancer, cancer has spread to nearby blood vessels and it may be in nearby lymph nodes and other tissues.
- The goal of treatment is to prevent or delay disease progression and to control the spread of disease.
- A clinical trial is preferred as first-line therapy for those with good performance status (PS) and for those with good PS with disease progression.
- Good PS is usually PS 0 or PS 1 with good biliary drainage and adequate nutritional intake.
- Poor PS is PS 2, PS 3, or PS 4. Those with poor PS may benefit from palliative and best supportive care with systemic therapy or palliative radiation therapy.
- Your care team will look for signs of disease progression and monitor your PS throughout treatment.
- Talk to your doctor about what you want from treatment. You can always decide not to continue with systemic therapy.

8 Metastatic

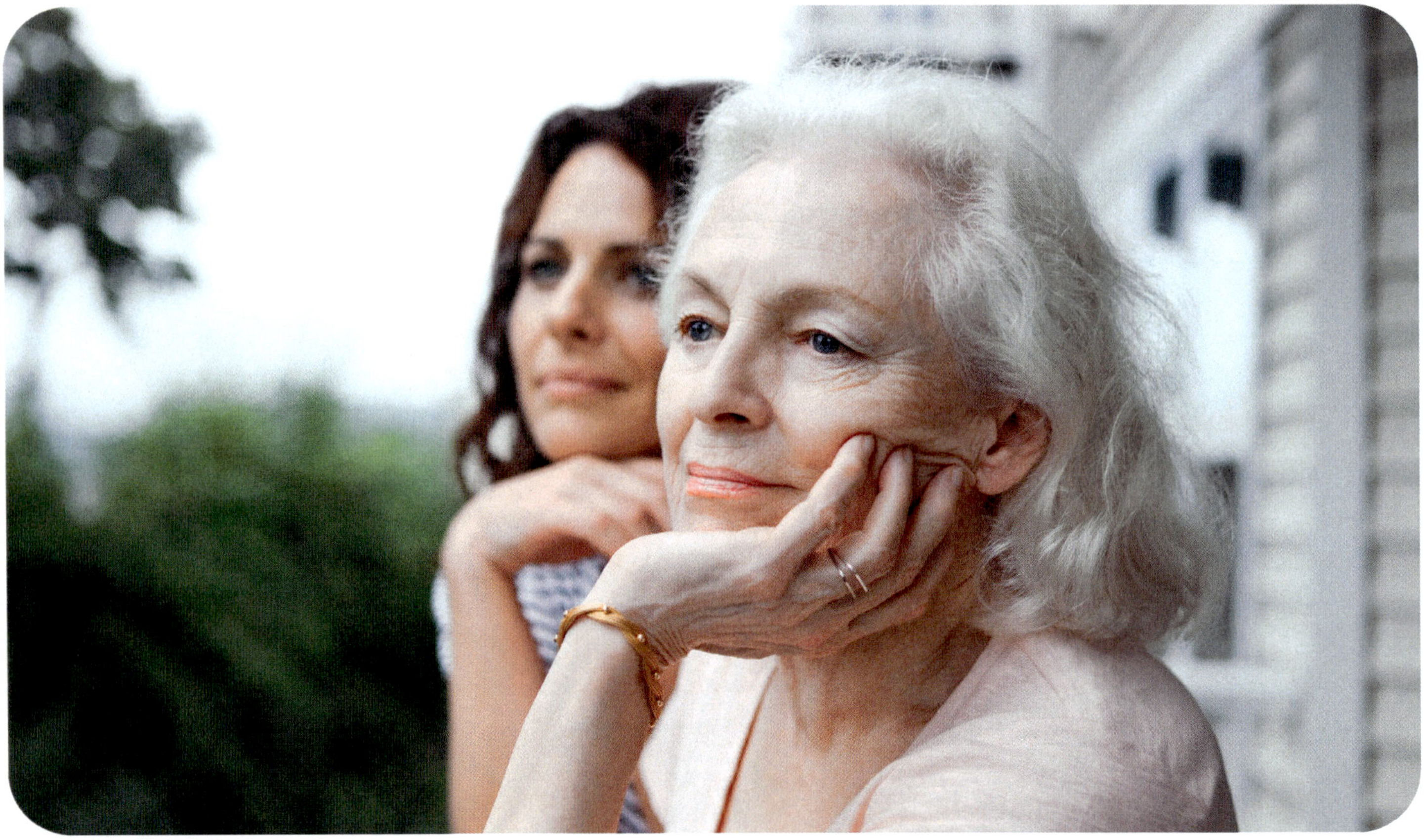

Metastatic cancer has spread to distant sites in the body. Together, you and your doctor will choose a treatment plan that is best for you.

Overview

Metastatic pancreatic cancer is cancer that has spread to distant sites in the body. Metastatic tumors are formed when cancer cells spread through the blood or lymphatic system to sites or organs that are far away from the pancreas. Metastatic pancreatic cancer is not treated with surgery.

The goals of metastatic pancreatic cancer treatment include symptom relief, quality of life, and longer survival.

Before treatment

Before treatment starts, you will be treated for jaundice. Jaundice is caused by a blocked bile duct. A stent will be placed unless a biliary bypass was performed earlier.

Genetic (germline) testing is recommended for anyone with confirmed pancreatic cancer. It looks for hereditary cancer syndromes which are those inherited from your parents.

Biomarker (tumor) testing is recommended for those who are candidates for anti-cancer therapy. It is used to identify uncommon mutations that can inform treatment decisions.

Guide 15
First-line systemic therapy options: Metastatic disease with good PS

Preferred options	• FOLFIRINOX or modified FOLFIRINOX • Gemcitabine with albumin-bound paclitaxel
	Only for known *BRCA1, BRCA2,* or *PALB2* mutations: • FOLFIRINOX or modified FOLFIRINOX • Gemcitabine with cisplatin
Other recommended	• Gemcitabine with erlotinib • Gemcitabine • Gemcitabine with capecitabine • Fixed-dose-rate gemcitabine, docetaxel, capecitabine (GTX regimen) • Fluoropyrimidine with oxaliplatin

First-line therapy

First-line treatment is the first treatment or set of treatments given to control the cancer. It is based on performance status (PS).

Good PS

Good PS is usually PS 0 or PS 1 with good biliary drainage and adequate nutritional intake. Good PS is treated with a clinical trial (preferred) or systemic therapy. Systemic therapy options are found in Guide 15.

Poor PS

Poor PS is PS 2, PS 3, or PS 4. Palliative and best supportive care are always given for those with poor PS. Chemotherapy or targeted therapy might be options based on genetic and tumor tests. Palliative radiation might be given.

Systemic therapy options for poor PS include gemcitabine, capecitabine, or continuous infusion 5-FU.

In some cases, pembrolizumab (only for MSI-H or dMMR tumors), larotrectinib (if *NTRK* gene fusion-positive), or entrectinib (if *NTRK* gene fusion-positive) might be used.

Maintenance therapy

Those who have good PS and stable disease after at least 4 to 6 months of chemotherapy may undergo maintenance therapy. Maintenance therapy might be a continuation of your current systemic therapy, but at a lower dose. A chemotherapy holiday is another option. A clinical trial or other systemic therapy options are also available.

Maintenance therapy options can be found in Guide 16.

Guide 16
Maintenance therapy options: Metastatic disease

Preferred options	If previous platinum-based chemotherapy: • Olaparib (only for germline *BRCA1 or BRCA2* mutations)
Other recommended	Clinical trial
	If previous first-line FOLFIRINOX: Capecitabine
	If previous first-line gemcitabine with nab-paclitaxel: • Gemcitabine with nab-paclitaxel modified schedule • Gemcitabine single agent
Used in some cases	If previous first-line FOLFIRINOX: • 5-FU with or without irinotecan • FOLFOX

Disease progression

If first-line treatment doesn't stop the cancer from growing, then a second-line treatment might be an option. Second-line treatment is the next set of treatments given to control the cancer when the first or previous treatments failed to stop cancer growth. It is based on your performance status (PS).

Second-line therapy will be a different systemic therapy than before. It is possible to have multiple lines of therapy. Talk with your doctor about what you want from treatment. You can always decide not to continue with systemic therapy. See Guide 17.

Guide 17
Second-line therapy options: Metastatic disease with good PS

If you had gemcitabine-based therapy before	• 5-FU with leucovorin and liposomal irinotecan • 5-FU with leucovorin and irinotecan (FOLFIRI) • FOLFIRINOX or modified FOLFIRINOX • Oxaliplatin with 5-FU and leucovorin (OFF) • FOLFOX • Capecitabine with oxaliplatin • Capecitabine • Continuous infusion 5-FU
If you had fluoropyrimidine-based therapy before	• Gemcitabine • Gemcitabine with albumin-bound paclitaxel • Gemcitabine with cisplatin (only for known *BRCA1, BRCA2,* or *PALB2* mutations) • Gemcitabine with erlotinib • 5-FU with leucovorin and liposomal irinotecan (if no prior irinotecan)
Used in some cases	• Pembrolizumab (only for MSI-H or dMMR tumors) • Larotrectinib (if *NTRK* gene fusion-positive) • Entrectinib (if *NTRK* gene fusion-positive)

Poor PS

If your PS is poor, then you may benefit from palliative and best supportive care with one of the following:

- Chemotherapy
- Targeted therapy
- Palliative RT for severe pain

Good PS

For good PS, treatment options are:

- Clinical trial (preferred)
- Systemic therapy or possibly targeted therapy
- Radiation therapy for severe pain

After second-line treatments, next steps would be palliative and best supportive care or clinical trial.

Get to know your care team and let them get to know you.

Review

- Metastatic pancreatic cancer is cancer that has spread to distant sites in the body.
- Metastatic pancreatic cancer is not treated with surgery.
- Before beginning treatment, your doctor will first treat symptoms such as jaundice.
- Genetic (germline) and biomarker (tumor) testing are recommended for those with confirmed metastatic disease. MSI and MMR testing are done usually as part of genetic or biomarker testing.
- A clinical trial is the preferred first-line treatment and second-line treatment option for those with good performance status (PS).
- Those with poor PS may benefit from palliative and best supportive care with systemic therapy or palliative radiation therapy.
- Talk to your doctor about what you want from treatment. You can always decide not to continue with systemic therapy.

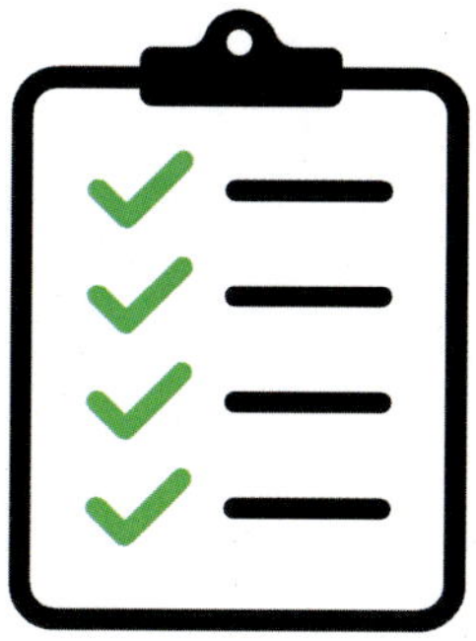

We want your feedback!

Our goal is to provide helpful and easy-to-understand information on cancer.

Take our survey to let us know what we got right and what we could do better:

NCCN.org/patients/feedback

9

Making treatment decisions

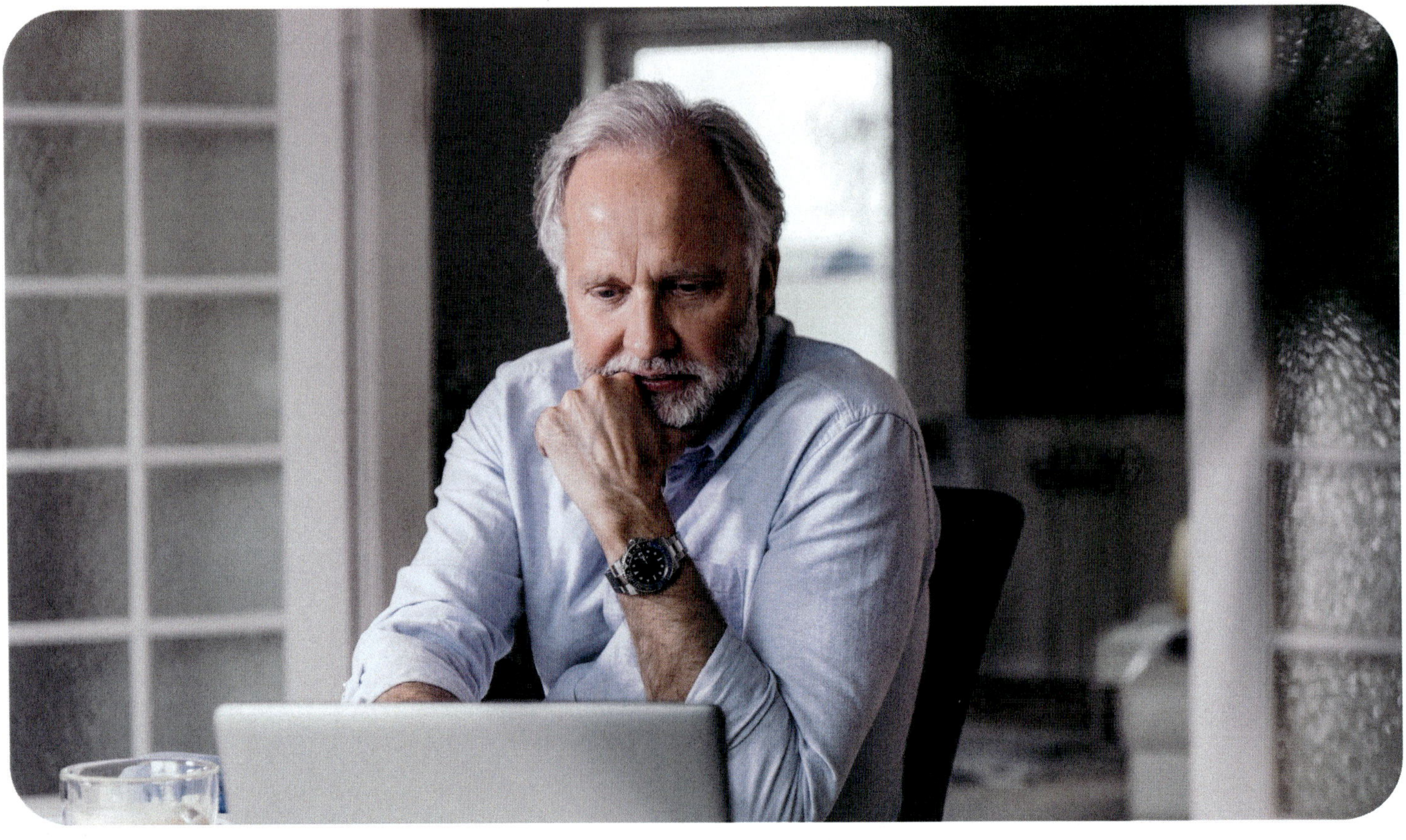

It's important to be comfortable with the cancer treatment you choose. This choice starts with having an open and honest conversation with your doctor.

It's your choice

In shared decision-making, you and your doctors share information, discuss the options, and agree on a treatment plan. It starts with an open and honest conversation between you and your doctor.

Treatment decisions are very personal. What is important to you may not be important to someone else.

Some things that may play a role in your decision-making:

- What you want and how that might differ from what others want
- Your religious and spiritual beliefs
- Your feelings about certain treatments like surgery or chemotherapy
- Your feelings about pain or side effects such as nausea and vomiting
- Cost of treatment, travel to treatment centers, and time away from school, family, or work
- Quality of life and length of life
- How active you are and the activities that are important to you

Think about what you want from treatment. Discuss openly the risks and benefits of specific treatments and procedures. Weigh options and share concerns with your doctor. If you take the time to build a relationship with your doctor, it will help you feel supported when considering options and making treatment decisions.

Second opinion

It is normal to want to start treatment as soon as possible. While cancer can't be ignored, there is time to have another doctor review your test results and suggest a treatment plan. This is called getting a second opinion, and it's a normal part of cancer care. Even doctors get second opinions!

Things you can do to prepare:

- Check with your insurance company about its rules on second opinions. There may be out-of-pocket costs to see doctors who are not part of your insurance plan.
- Make plans to have copies of all your records sent to the doctor you will see for your second opinion.

Support groups

Many people diagnosed with cancer find support groups to be helpful. Support groups often include people at different stages of treatment. If your hospital or community doesn't have support groups for people with cancer, check out the websites listed in this book.

Questions to ask your doctors

Possible questions to ask your doctors are listed on the following pages. Feel free to use these questions or come up with your own. Be clear about your goals for treatment and find out what to expect from treatment.

Questions to ask about testing and staging

1. What tests will I have? How often will they be repeated? Will my insurance pay for these tests?
2. When will I have a biopsy? Will I have more than one? What are the risks?
3. Will a stent be placed during my biopsy? What else might be done?
4. How soon will I know the results and who will explain them to me?
5. Who will talk with me about the next steps? When?
6. What genetic tests will I have for inherited or other mutations? When?
7. What will you do to make me comfortable during testing?
8. Is my cancer resectable, borderline resectable, or unresectable?
9. Is my cancer locally advanced or metastatic?
10. Is the cancer in any other organs like my liver, lungs, or bone?
11. What does my stage mean in terms of length of survival and quality of life?

Questions to ask your doctors about their experience

1. What is your experience treating pancreatic cancer?
2. What is the experience of those on your team?
3. Do you only treat pancreatic cancer? What else do you treat?
4. I would like to get a second opinion. Is there someone you recommend?
5. How many patients like me (of the same age, gender, race) have you treated?
6. Will you be consulting with experts to discuss my care? Who will you consult?
7. How many procedures like the one you're suggesting have you done?
8. Is this treatment a major part of your practice?
9. How many of your patients have had complications? What were the complications?
10. How many pancreatic cancer surgeries have you done?
11. Who will manage my day-to-day care?

Questions to ask about options

1. What will happen if I do nothing?
2. How do my age, overall health, and other factors affect the options?
3. Am I a candidate for a clinical trial?
4. Which option is proven to work best for my cancer, age, and other risk factors?
5. Does any option offer a long-term cancer control? Are the chances any better for one option than another? Less time-consuming? Less expensive?
6. Which treatment will give me the best quality of life? Which treatment will extend life? By how long?
7. What are our options if the treatment stops working?
8. Can I stop treatment at any time? What will happen if I stop treatment?
9. Is there a social worker or someone who can help me decide?
10. Is there a hospital or treatment center you can recommend? Can I go to one hospital for surgery and a different center for systemic or radiation therapy?

Questions to ask about treatment

1. What are my treatment choices? What are the benefits and risks? Which treatment do you recommend and why?
2. How will my age, performance status, cancer stage, and other health conditions limit my treatment choices?
3. Does the order of treatment matter?
4. How long do I have to decide about treatment?
5. Does this hospital or center offer the best treatment for me?
6. When will I start treatment? How long will treatment take? What should I wear to treatment?
7. How much will the treatment cost? How much will my insurance pay for?
8. What are the chances my cancer will return? How will it be treated if it returns?
9. I would like a second opinion. Is there someone you can recommend?
10. How will treatment affect my ability to digest food? Will I be able to do things I enjoy?

Questions to ask about surgery

1. If my cancer is resectable, how much of my tumor will be removed? How much of my pancreas will be removed?
2. What other organs or tissues might be removed during surgery? What will this mean in terms of my survival and recovery?
3. What kind of surgery will I have? Will it be open or minimally invasive? Will I have more than one surgery?
4. Does my cancer involve any veins or arteries? How might this affect surgery?
5. What are the chances you can remove the whole tumor and I will have a negative margin?
6. What happens if during surgery you find you can't remove the tumor?
7. How long will it take me to recover from surgery?
8. How much pain will I be in? What will be done to manage my pain?
9. What is the chance that this surgery will shorten my life?
10. What other side effects can I expect from surgery? What complications can occur from this surgery?
11. What treatment will I have before, during, or after surgery? What does this treatment do?
12. Will I need a stent?

Questions to ask about radiation therapy

1. What type of radiation therapy will I have?
2. What will you target?
3. What is the goal of this radiation treatment?
4. How many treatment sessions will I require? Can you do a shorter course of radiation?
5. Do you offer this type of radiation here? If not, can you refer me to someone who does?
6. What side effects can I expect from radiation?
7. What should I wear?

Questions to ask about side effects

1. What are the side effects of systemic therapy? Surgery? A stent? A biliary bypass?
2. What are the side effects of pancreatic cancer?
3. How long will these side effects last? Do any side effects lessen or worsen in severity over time?
4. What side effects should I watch for? What side effects are expected and which are life threatening?
5. When should I call the doctor? Can I text? What should I do on weekends and other non-office hours?
6. What emergency department or ER should I go to? Will my treatment team be able to communicate with the ER team?
7. What medicines can I take to prevent or relieve side effects?
8. What can I do to help with pain and other side effects?
9. Will you stop treatment or change treatment if there are side effects? What do you look for?
10. What can I do to lessen or prevent side effects? What will you do?
11. What medicines may worsen side effects of treatment?

Questions to ask about clinical trials

1. What clinical trials are available for my type and stage of pancreatic cancer?
2. What are the treatments used in the clinical trial?
3. What does the treatment do?
4. Has the treatment been used before? Has it been used for other types of cancer?
5. What are the risks and benefits of this treatment?
6. What side effects should I expect? How will the side effects be controlled?
7. How long will I be in the clinical trial?
8. Will I be able to get other treatment if this doesn't work?
9. How will I know if the treatment is working?
10. Will the clinical trial cost me anything? If so, how much?

Resources

American Association for Clinical Chemistry
labtestsonline.org

American Cancer Society
cancer.org/cancer/pancreatic-cancer.html

cancer.org/content/dam/cancer-org/cancer-control/en/worksheets/pain-diary.pdf

Cancer*Care*
cancercare.org

Chemocare
chemocare.com

Hirshberg Foundation for Pancreatic Cancer Research
pancreatic.org

Let's Win! Pancreatic Cancer Foundation
letswinpc.org

Lustgarten Foundation for Pancreatic Cancer Research
lustgarten.org

MedlinePlus
medlineplus.gov

My Survival Story
mysurvivalstory.org

National Cancer Institute
cancer.gov/types/pancreatic

National Hospice and Palliative Care Organization
nhpco.org/patients-and-caregivers

OncoLink
oncolink.org

Pancreatic Cancer Action Network (PanCAN)
pancan.org

clinicaltrials.pancan.org

Radiological Society of North America
radiologyinfo.org

The National Pancreas Foundation
pancreasfoundation.org

animatedpancreaspatient.com/en-pancreas/home

World Pancreatic Cancer Coalition
worldpancreaticcancercoalition.org

share with us.

Take our survey
And help make the NCCN Guidelines for Patients better for everyone!

NCCN.org/patients/comments

Words to know

adjuvant
Treatment given after the main treatment used to rid the body of cancer.

best supportive care
Treatment to improve quality of life and relieve discomfort.

bile duct
A tiny tube or vessel in the body that drains digestive fluid (bile) from the liver.

biliary bypass
Surgery to re-route the flow of bile, digestive fluid, from the common bile duct into the small intestine.

biliary stent
A small plastic or metal tube-shaped device used to unblock a bile duct.

bilirubin
A yellow-brown substance that is removed from blood by the liver and is part of bile.

borderline resectable
Cancer that is confined to the pancreas but approaches nearby structures or has severe symptoms, raising concern that it might or might not be possible to remove all the cancer with surgery.

CA 19-9
Proteins made by cancer cells and found in blood.

celiac plexus neurolysis
Ethanol is injected into the nerves of the abdomen to block pain.

chemoradiation
Treatment that combines chemotherapy and radiation therapy.

chemotherapy
Drugs that kill fast-growing cells throughout the body, including cancer cells and normal cells.

cholangitis
An infection of the bile ducts that drain digestive fluids out of the liver.

common bile duct
A tiny tube that carries digestive fluid (bile) from the liver into the small intestine, which absorbs nutrients from eaten food.

computed tomography (CT)
A test that uses x-rays from many angles to make a picture of the inside of the body.

contrast
A chemical put into your body to make clearer pictures during imaging tests.

core needle biopsy
A procedure that removes tissue samples with a hollow needle. Also called core biopsy.

CT-guided FNA biopsy
Use of pictures from a CT (computed tomography) scan to guide a thin needle to the right spot to remove a sample of tissue from the body for testing.

distal pancreatectomy
Surgery that removes the widest part (body) and narrow end (tail) of the pancreas as well as other nearby organs.

ductal adenocarcinoma
Cancer of the cells that line the pancreatic ducts and small tubes that fluids pass through, and make proteins that digest food.

duodenal bypass
Surgery to re-route the path that eaten food takes from the stomach to the small intestine, which absorbs nutrients from food.

endoscopic retrograde cholangiopancreatography (ERCP)
A test that uses x-rays and a thin, lighted tube that is inserted into the body to see the pancreatic ducts and bile ducts.

endoscopic ultrasound (EUS)
A test that uses a thin, lighted tube guided through the mouth and down the throat to take pictures of the inside of the body using sound waves.

EUS-guided FNA biopsy
Use of pictures from sound waves and a thin, lighted tube inserted through the mouth to guide a thin needle to the right spot to remove a sample of tissue from the body for testing. Also called EUS-FNA.

fine-needle aspiration (FNA) or fine-needle biopsy (FNB)
Use of a thin needle to remove a small amount of tissue or fluid from the body to test for cancer cells.

first-line treatment
The first drug or set of drugs given to treat a disease. Might be followed by second-line or more lines of treatment.

fluoropyrimidine-based therapy
A combination chemotherapy regimen in which the main drug used is 5-FU (5-fluorouracil).

FOLFIRINOX
A combination chemotherapy regimen that includes 5-FU, leucovorin, irinotecan, and oxaliplatin.

FOLFOX
A combination chemotherapy regimen that includes 5-FU, leucovorin, and oxaliplatin.

gastroenterologist
A doctor who's an expert in diseases of the digestive system. This system contains organs that break down food for the body to use.

gastrojejunostomy
Surgery to bypass a blockage in the part of the stomach that empties into the small intestine.

gemcitabine-based therapy
A combination chemotherapy regimen in which the main drug used is gemcitabine.

gene
Coded instructions in cells for making new cells and controlling how cells behave.

hereditary
Passed down from parent to child through coded information in cells (genes).

immunotherapy
A treatment with drugs that help the body find and destroy cancer cells.

interventional radiologist
A doctor who is an expert in imaging tests and using image-guided tools to perform minimally invasive techniques to diagnose or treat disease.

jaundice
Yellowing of the skin and eyes due to a buildup of bilirubin in the body.

laparoscopy
A surgical test that uses a thin, lighted tube inserted through a small cut in the belly (abdomen) to see inside the belly area and possibly remove tissue for testing.

liver function test
A blood test that measures chemicals that are made or processed by the liver to check how well the liver is working.

locally advanced pancreatic cancer
Cancer that started in the pancreas and has grown into nearby blood vessels or tissues.

local recurrence
Cancer that came back after treatment. Found in or near the pancreas.

magnetic resonance cholangiopancreatography (MRCP)
A test that uses radio waves and powerful magnets to make very clear pictures of the pancreas and bile ducts.

magnetic resonance imaging (MRI)
A test that uses radio waves and powerful magnets to make pictures of the inside of the body showing the shape and function of body parts.

main pancreatic duct
A small tube in the body that drains digestive fluids from the pancreas into the first part of the small intestine (duodenum).

medical oncologist
A doctor who is an expert in cancer drugs.

metastasectomy
Surgery to remove a metastasis.

metastasis
Cancer that has spread from the first tumor to another body part. Can be local (near the primary tumor) or distant.

monitoring
Testing after treatment ends to check for the return of cancer. Also called surveillance.

neoadjuvant
The treatment given before the main (primary) treatment used to rid the body of cancer.

oncologist
A doctor who is an expert in the treatment of cancer.

palliative care
Health care that includes symptom relief but not cancer treatment. Also sometimes called supportive care.

palliative radiation
Radiation used to relieve symptoms such as pain caused by pancreatic cancer or cancer treatment.

pancreatic duct
A small tube in the pancreas that digestive fluids pass through.

pancreatic protocol CT
A CT scan that is done in a certain way so that all of the pictures focus specifically on the pancreas to clearly show the pancreas, nearby blood vessels, and very tiny tumors elsewhere in your abdomen.

pancreatoduodenectomy
Surgery to remove the widest part (head) of the pancreas and parts of other nearby organs. Also called Whipple procedure.

pathologist
A doctor who is an expert in testing cells and tissue to find disease.

percutaneous endoscopic gastrostomy (PEG) tube
A tube inserted through a cut in the abdomen and placed into the stomach to give food.

performance status (PS)
A rating of a person's symptoms and ability to do daily activities.

positron emission tomography (PET)
A test that uses two picture-making methods to show the shape and function of tissue.

primary treatment
The main treatment used to rid the body of cancer. In resectable pancreatic cancer, surgery is the primary treatment.

radiation therapy (RT)
The use of high-energy rays (radiation) to destroy cancer cells.

recurrence
The return of cancer after treatment. Also called relapse.

resectable
Cancer that can be completely removed with surgery.

stereotactic body radiation therapy (SBRT)
Radiation therapy given in higher doses to smaller areas over 1 to 5 sessions of treatment.

superior mesenteric artery
The large, tube-shaped vessel that carries blood from the heart to the intestines—the organ food passes through after leaving the stomach.

superior mesenteric vein
The large, tube-shaped vessel that returns blood from the intestines—organ food passes through after leaving the stomach—back to the heart.

supportive care
Treatment given to relieve symptoms caused by cancer or cancer treatment. Also called palliative care.

surgical margin
The normal-looking tissue around the edge of the tumor removed during surgery.

surveillance
Testing to watch for cancer growth. No treatment is given during this time.

total pancreatectomy
Surgery to remove the entire pancreas and other nearby organs and tissues.

unresectable
Cancer that can't be removed by surgery.

Whipple procedure
Surgery to remove the head of the pancreas and parts of other nearby organs. Also called pancreaticoduodenectomy.

NCCN Contributors

This patient guide is based on the NCCN Clinical Practice Guidelines in Oncology (NCCN Guidelines®) for Pancreatic Cancer, Version 2.2021. It was adapted, reviewed, and published with help from the following people:

Dorothy A. Shead, MS
Senior Director
Patient Information Operations

Rachael Clarke
Senior Medical Copyeditor

Tanya Fischer, MEd, MSLIS
Medical Writer

Laura J. Hanisch, PsyD
Medical Writer/Patient Information Specialist

Stephanie Helbling, MPH, CHES®
Medical Writer

Susan Kidney
Graphic Design Specialist

John Murphy
Medical Writer

Erin Vidic, MA
Medical Writer

Kim Williams
Creative Services Manager

NCCN Clinical Practice Guidelines in Oncology (NCCN Guidelines®) for Pancreatic Cancer, Version 2.2021 were developed by the following NCCN Panel Members:

Margaret A. Tempero, MD/Chair
UCSF Helen Diller Family Comprehensive Cancer Center

Mokenge P. Malafa, MD/Vice Chair
Moffitt Cancer Center

*Mahmoud Al-Hawary, MD
University of Michigan Rogel Cancer Center

*Stephen W. Behrman, MD
The University of Tennessee Health Science Center

Al B. Benson III, MD
Robert H. Lurie Comprehensive Cancer Center of Northwestern University

Dana B. Cardin, MD
Vanderbilt-Ingram Cancer Center

*E. Gabriela Chiorean, MD
Fred Hutchinson Cancer Research Center/Seattle Cancer Care Alliance

Vincent Chung, MD
City of Hope National Medical Center

Brian Czito, MD
Duke Cancer Institute

Marco Del Chiaro, MD, PhD
University of Colorado Cancer Center

Mary Dillhoff, MD
The Ohio State University Comprehensive Cancer Center -James Cancer Hospital and Solove Research Institute

Timothy R. Donahue, MD
UCLA Jonsson Comprehensive Cancer Center

Efrat Dotan, MD
Fox Chase Cancer Center

Cristina R. Ferrone, MD
Massachusetts General Hospital Cancer Center

Christos Fountzilas, MD
Roswell Park Comprehensive Cancer Center

Jeffrey Hardacre, MD
Case Comprehensive Cancer Center/University Hospitals Seidman Cancer Center and Cleveland Clinic Taussig Cancer Institute

William G. Hawkins, MD
Siteman Cancer Center at Barnes-Jewish Hospital and Washington University School of Medicine

Kelsey Klute, MD
Fred & Pamela Buffett Cancer Center

Andrew H. Ko, MD
UCSF Helen Diller Family Comprehensive Cancer Center

John W. Kunstman, MD, MHS
Yale Cancer Center/ Smilow Cancer Hospital

Noelle LoConte, MD
University of Wisconsin Carbone Cancer Center

Andrew M. Lowy, MD
UC San Diego Moores Cancer Center

*Cassadie Moravek
Pancreatic Cancer Action Network

Eric K. Nakakura, MD
UCSF Helen Diller Family Comprehensive Cancer Center

Amol K. Narang, MD
The Sidney Kimmel Comprehensive Cancer Center at Johns Hopkins

Jorge Obando, MD
Duke Cancer Institute

*Patricio M. Polanco, MD
UT Southwestern Simmons Comprehensive Cancer Center

Sushanth Reddy, MD
O'Neal Comprehensive Cancer Center at UAB

Marsha Reyngold, MD, PhD
Memorial Sloan Kettering Cancer Center

Courtney Scaife, MD
Huntsman Cancer Institute at the University of Utah

Jeanne Shen, MD
Stanford Cancer Institute

Charles Vollmer Jr., MD
Abramson Cancer Center at the University of Pennsylvania

Robert A. Wolff, MD
The University of Texas MD Anderson Cancer Center

Brian M. Wolpin, MD, MPH
Dana-Farber/Brigham and Women's Cancer Center

NCCN Staff

Beth Lynn RN, BS, CMSRN
Guidelines Layout Specialist

Giby George, MD
Oncology Scientist/Medical Writer

* Reviewed this patient guide. For disclosures, visit NCCN.org/disclosures.

NCCN Cancer Centers

Abramson Cancer Center
at the University of Pennsylvania
Philadelphia, Pennsylvania
800.789.7366 • pennmedicine.org/cancer

Fred & Pamela Buffett Cancer Center
Omaha, Nebraska
402.559.5600 • unmc.edu/cancercenter

Case Comprehensive Cancer Center/
University Hospitals Seidman Cancer
Center and Cleveland Clinic Taussig
Cancer Institute
Cleveland, Ohio
800.641.2422 • UH Seidman Cancer Center
uhhospitals.org/services/cancer-services
866.223.8100 • CC Taussig Cancer Institute
my.clevelandclinic.org/departments/cancer
216.844.8797 • Case CCC
case.edu/cancer

City of Hope National Medical Center
Los Angeles, California
800.826.4673 • cityofhope.org

Dana-Farber/Brigham and
Women's Cancer Center |
Massachusetts General Hospital
Cancer Center
Boston, Massachusetts
617.732.5500
youhaveus.org
617.726.5130
massgeneral.org/cancer-center

Duke Cancer Institute
Durham, North Carolina
888.275.3853 • dukecancerinstitute.org

Fox Chase Cancer Center
Philadelphia, Pennsylvania
888.369.2427 • foxchase.org

Huntsman Cancer Institute
at the University of Utah
Salt Lake City, Utah
800.824.2073
huntsmancancer.org

Fred Hutchinson Cancer
Research Center/Seattle
Cancer Care Alliance
Seattle, Washington
206.606.7222 • seattlecca.org
206.667.5000 • fredhutch.org

The Sidney Kimmel Comprehensive
Cancer Center at Johns Hopkins
Baltimore, Maryland
410.955.8964
www.hopkinskimmelcancercenter.org

Robert H. Lurie Comprehensive
Cancer Center of Northwestern
University
Chicago, Illinois
866.587.4322 • cancer.northwestern.edu

Mayo Clinic Cancer Center
Phoenix/Scottsdale, Arizona
Jacksonville, Florida
Rochester, Minnesota
480.301.8000 • Arizona
904.953.0853 • Florida
507.538.3270 • Minnesota
mayoclinic.org/cancercenter

Memorial Sloan Kettering
Cancer Center
New York, New York
800.525.2225 • mskcc.org

Moffitt Cancer Center
Tampa, Florida
888.663.3488 • moffitt.org

The Ohio State University
Comprehensive Cancer Center -
James Cancer Hospital and
Solove Research Institute
Columbus, Ohio
800.293.5066 • cancer.osu.edu

O'Neal Comprehensive
Cancer Center at UAB
Birmingham, Alabama
800.822.0933 • uab.edu/onealcancercenter

Roswell Park Comprehensive
Cancer Center
Buffalo, New York
877.275.7724 • roswellpark.org

Siteman Cancer Center at Barnes-
Jewish Hospital and Washington
University School of Medicine
St. Louis, Missouri
800.600.3606 • siteman.wustl.edu

St. Jude Children's Research Hospital/
The University of Tennessee
Health Science Center
Memphis, Tennessee
866.278.5833 • stjude.org
901.448.5500 • uthsc.edu

Stanford Cancer Institute
Stanford, California
877.668.7535 • cancer.stanford.edu

UC Davis
Comprehensive Cancer Center
Sacramento, California
916.734.5959 | 800.770.9261
health.ucdavis.edu/cancer

UC San Diego Moores Cancer Center
La Jolla, California
858.822.6100 • cancer.ucsd.edu

UCLA Jonsson
Comprehensive Cancer Center
Los Angeles, California
310.825.5268 • cancer.ucla.edu

UCSF Helen Diller Family
Comprehensive Cancer Center
San Francisco, California
800.689.8273 • cancer.ucsf.edu

University of Colorado Cancer Center
Aurora, Colorado
720.848.0300 • coloradocancercenter.org

University of Michigan
Rogel Cancer Center
Ann Arbor, Michigan
800.865.1125 • rogelcancercenter.org

The University of Texas
MD Anderson Cancer Center
Houston, Texas
844.269.5922 • mdanderson.org

University of Wisconsin
Carbone Cancer Center
Madison, Wisconsin
608.265.1700 • uwhealth.org/cancer

UT Southwestern Simmons
Comprehensive Cancer Center
Dallas, Texas
214.648.3111 • utsouthwestern.edu/simmons

Vanderbilt-Ingram Cancer Center
Nashville, Tennessee
877.936.8422 • vicc.org

Yale Cancer Center/
Smilow Cancer Hospital
New Haven, Connecticut
855.4.SMILOW • yalecancercenter.org

Index

Made in the USA
Coppell, TX
18 February 2023

13000956R00057